50 Studies Every Palliative Care
Doctor Should Know

50 STUDIES EVERY DOCTOR SHOULD KNOW

50 Studies Every Doctor Should Know: The Key Studies that Form
the Foundation of Evidence-Based Medicine, Revised Edition
Michael E. Hochman

50 Studies Every Internist Should Know
*Kristopher Swiger, Joshua R. Thomas, Michael E. Hochman,
and Steven Hochman*

50 Studies Every Neurologist Should Know
David Y. Hwang and David M. Greer

50 Studies Every Pediatrician Should Know
*Ashaunta T. Anderson, Nina L. Shapiro, Stephen C. Aronoff,
Jeremiah Davis, and Michael Levy*

50 Imaging Studies Every Doctor Should Know
Christoph I. Lee

50 Studies Every Surgeon Should Know
SreyRam Kuy, Rachel J. Kwon, and Miguel A. Burch

50 Studies Every Intensivist Should Know
Edward A. Bittner

50 Studies Every Palliative Care Doctor Should Know
David Hui, Akhila Reddy, and Eduardo Bruera

50 Studies Every Psychiatrist Should Know
Ish P. Bhalla, Rajesh R. Tampi, and Vinod H. Srihari

50 Studies Every Palliative Care Doctor Should Know

EDITED BY

DAVID HUI, MD, MSc
Associate Professor
Department of Palliative, Rehabilitation, and Integrative Medicine
The University of Texas MD Anderson Cancer Center
Houston, TX

AKHILA REDDY, MD
Associate Professor
Department of Palliative, Rehabilitation, and Integrative Medicine
The University of Texas MD Anderson Cancer Center
Houston, TX

EDUARDO BRUERA, MD
F.T. McGraw Chair in the Treatment of Cancer
Chair, Department of Palliative, Rehabilitation, and Integrative Medicine
The University of Texas MD Anderson Cancer Center
Houston, TX

SERIES EDITOR

MICHAEL E. HOCHMAN, MD, MPH
Assistant Professor, Medicine
Director, Gehr Family Center for Implementation Science
USC Keck School of Medicine
Los Angeles, CA

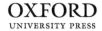

OXFORD
UNIVERSITY PRESS

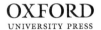

UNIVERSITY PRESS

Oxford University Press is a department of the University of Oxford. It furthers
the University's objective of excellence in research, scholarship, and education
by publishing worldwide. Oxford is a registered trade mark of Oxford University
Press in the UK and certain other countries.

Published in the United States of America by Oxford University Press
198 Madison Avenue, New York, NY 10016, United States of America.

Library of Congress Cataloging-in-Publication Data
Names: Hui, David, 1975– editor. | Reddy, Akhila, editor. | Bruera, Eduardo, editor.
Title: 50 studies every palliative care doctor should know /
edited by David Hui, Akhila Reddy, Eduardo Bruera.
Other titles: Fifty studies every palliative doctor should know |
50 studies every doctor should know (Series)
Description: Oxford ; New York : Oxford University Press, [2018] |
Series: 50 studies every doctor should know
Identifiers: LCCN 2017042098 | ISBN 9780190658618 (pbk. : alk. paper)
Subjects: | MESH: Palliative Care | Evidence-Based Medicine | Clinical Trials as Topic
Classification: LCC R726.8 | NLM WB 310 | DDC 616.02/9—dc23
LC record available at https://lccn.loc.gov/2017042098

9 8 7 6 5 4

Printed by Marquis, Canada

To Nancy
David Hui

To my wonderful parents, Drs. Lakshman Reddy and Prathibha Devi
Akhila Reddy

To Sebastian
Eduardo Bruera

CONTENTS

SECTION 2   Symptom Assessment and Management

PREFACE

Over the past five decades, palliative care has evolved from serving patients at the end of life into a highly specialized discipline focused on delivering supportive care to patients with life-limiting illnesses throughout the disease trajectory. A growing body of evidence is now available to inform the key domains in the practice of palliative care, including symptom management, psychosocial care, communication, decision-making, and end-of-life care. Findings from multiple studies indicate that integrating palliative care early in the disease trajectory can result in improvements in quality of life, symptom control, patient and caregiver satisfaction and knowledge of the disease, quality of end-of-life care, survival, and costs of care.

Building on the successful series *50 Studies Every Doctor Should Know*, this title aims to provide a concise, up-to-date, and clear summary of the landmark studies that have significantly advanced our understanding of palliative care–related-issues and transformed clinical practice. Our list of potential studies includes randomized controlled trials, major prospective observational studies, and a few systematic reviews. This book may be useful for practicing clinicians and trainees from many areas of medicine (e.g., palliative care, internal medicine, oncology, nephrology, cardiology, pulmonology, surgery, and gynecology) interested in learning more about the evidence to support practice in palliative care. It can also be a quick reference for researchers interested in reviewing the designs, outcomes, strengths, and weaknesses of major studies.

The 50 studies included here are based on a consensus among the editors and book reviewers. Admittedly, there are many more great studies than what we can include, and many more well-designed studies are being published every year. In selecting the 50 studies, several unique aspects of palliative care were taken into consideration. The practice of palliative care covers a wide range of topics across multiple disease types (e.g., cancer, heart failure, and dementia) and disciplines (e.g., medicine, nursing, psychology, and chaplaincy). In contrast to other more established medical specialties, the evidence base for palliative care is still evolving. Thus there are fewer randomized controlled trials. Moreover, many important issues relevant to the practice of palliative care cannot be addressed with randomized controlled trials scientifically, ethnically, or logistically. Observational studies can contribute to our knowledge, and some are practice-changing. We believe these timeless pieces all contribute to our practice and understanding of palliative care. We also strive to polish this list in future editions.

We would like to thank all the chapter authors, who are thought-leaders in this field, for their enormous contributions to this book. These experts have generously shared their knowledge, insights, and time to provide a balanced discussion of each study, putting the findings in the clinical context. We have reached out to the original study authors, whenever possible, to ensure proper reporting and interpretation.

We would like to thank Dr. Michael Hochman for his vision in creating this series. We are also grateful to Ms. Rebecca Suzan and Ms. Tiffany Lu from Oxford University Press for their editorial support and guidance. We would also like to express our gratitude to Ms. Sarai Portal for her unyielding support for this project.

David Hui, MD, MSc
Akhila Reddy, MD
Eduardo Bruera, MD

CONTRIBUTORS

Claudio Adile, MD
Pain Relief and Supportive Care Unit
La Maddalena Cancer Center
Palermo, Italy

Rajiv Agarwal, MD
Medical Oncology Fellow
Memorial Sloan Kettering
    Cancer Center
New York, NY

Joseph Arthur, MD
Associate Professor
Department of Palliative,
    Rehabilitation, and Integrative
    Medicine
Division of Cancer Medicine
The University of Texas MD
    Anderson Cancer Center
Houston, TX

Rebecca Burke, MD
Fellow, Hospice and Palliative Medicine
Department of Palliative,
    Rehabilitation, and Integrative
    Medicine
The University of Texas MD
    Anderson Cancer Center
Division of Cancer Medicine
Houston, TX

Shalini Dalal, MD
Associate Professor
Department of Palliative,
    Rehabilitation, and Integrative
    Medicine
The University of Texas MD
    Anderson Cancer Center
Division of Cancer Medicine
Houston, TX

Maxine de la Cruz, MD
Associate Professor
Department of Palliative,
    Rehabilitation, and Integrative
    Medicine
The University of Texas MD
    Anderson Cancer Center
Division of Cancer Medicine
Houston, TX

Marvin Omar Delgado-Guay, MD
Associate Professor
Department of Palliative,
    Rehabilitation, and Integrative
    Medicine
The University of Texas MD
    Anderson Cancer Center
Division of Cancer Medicine
Houston, TX

Anjali Varma Desai, MD
Palliative Medicine Fellow
Supportive Care Service
Memorial Sloan Kettering Cancer
    Center
New York, NY

Rony Dev, DO
Associate Professor
Department of Palliative,
    Rehabilitation, and Integrative
    Medicine
The University of Texas MD
    Anderson Cancer Center
Division of Cancer Medicine
Houston, TX

**André Filipe Junqueira dos Santos,
MD, PhD**
Coordinator, Palliative Care Unit
Clinics Hospital of Ribeirão Preto
University of São Paulo
Vice President
National Academy of Palliative Care
São Paulo, Brazil

Andrew S. Epstein, MD
Assistant Attending
Memorial Sloan Kettering
    Cancer Center
Gastrointestinal Oncology Service
Supportive Care Service
New York, NY

Esmé Finlay, MD
Associate Professor
Division of Palliative Medicine
Department of Internal Medicine
University of New Mexico School
    of Medicine
Albuquerque, NM

Erin FitzGerald, DO
Assistant Professor
Attending Physician Palliative
    Medicine
University of New Mexico School
    of Medicine
Albuquerque, NM

Lynn A. Flint, MD
Associate Professor
Division of Geriatrics
University of California,
    San Francisco
San Francisco, CA

Nathan A. Gray, MD
Assistant Professor
Duke University School of Medicine
Durham, NC

**Breffni Hannon, MB BCh BAO,
BMedSci, MMedSci, MCFP**
Palliative Care Physician
Princess Margaret Cancer Centre
Toronto, ON, Canada

Allison E. Jordan, MD, HMDC
Medical Director of Palliative
    Care Services
Christian and Alton Memorial
    Hospital
Associate Medical Director,
    BJC Hospice
St. Louis, MO

Arif H. Kamal, MD, MBA, MHS
Associate Professor of Medicine and
    Business Administration
Duke School of Medicine and Fuqua
    School of Business
Duke University
Durham, NC

Yu Jung Kim, MD, PhD
Associate Professor
Division of Hematology and Medical
   Oncology
Comprehensive Cancer Center
Department of Internal Medicine
Seoul National University Bundang
   Hospital
Seongnam, Republic of Korea

**Peter Lawlor, MB, FRCPI,
CCFP, MMedSc**
Associate Professor, Division of
   Palliative Care
Department of Medicine, University
   of Ottawa
Clinical Investigator, Bruyère
   and Ottawa Hospital Research
   Institutes
Physician, Palliative Care Unit,
   Bruyère Continuing Care
Ottawa, ON, Canada

**Thomas W. LeBlanc, MD, MA,
MHS, FAAHPM**
Associate Professor, Division of
   Hematologic Malignancies and
   Cellular Therapy
Department of Medicine, Duke
   University School of Medicine
Cancer Control and Population
   Sciences Program, Duke Cancer
   Institute
Durham, NC

Francisco Loaiciga, MD
Fellow, Hospice and Palliative
   Medicine
Department of Palliative,
   Rehabilitation, and Integrative
   Medicine
The University of Texas MD
   Anderson Cancer Center
Division of Cancer Medicine
Houston, TX

Regina Mackey, MD
Fellow, Hospice and Palliative
   Medicine
Department of Palliative,
   Rehabilitation, and Integrative
   Medicine
The University of Texas MD
   Anderson Cancer Center
Division of Cancer Medicine
Houston, TX

Emily Jean Martin, MD
Hospice and Palliative Medicine
   Fellow
University of California, San Diego
La Jolla, CA

Dutt Mehta, MD
Fellow, Hospice and Palliative
   Medicine
University of California, Los Angeles/
   Veterans Affairs Hospice and
   Palliative Care
Los Angeles, CA

Masanori Mori, MD
Palliative Care Team
Seirei Mikatahara General Hospital
Hamamatsu, Japan

Linh Nguyen, MD
Assistant Professor of Palliative
    Medicine
Department of Internal Medicine/
    Division of Geriatric and Palliative
    Medicine
The University of Texas McGovern
    Medical School
Houston, TX

Oreofe O. Odejide, MD, MPH
Division of Hematologic Malignances
Dana-Farber Cancer Institute
Instructor in Medicine
Harvard Medical School
Boston, MA

Lori Olson, MD
Assistant Professor
University of Kansas Medical Center
Kansas City, KS

Diaa Osman, DO, MPH
Hematology/Oncology Fellow
Department of Internal Medicine
University of New Mexico
    Cancer Center
Camino de Salud, NM

Carlos Eduardo Paiva, MD, PhD
Department of Clinical Oncology
Barretos Cancer Hospital
Barretos, Sao Paulo, Brazil

Ravi B. Parikh, MD
Fellow, Hematology and Oncology
Perelman School of Medicine
University of Pennsylvania
Philadelphia, PA

Chirag A. Patel, MD
Taussig Cancer Institute,
Section of Palliative Medicine and
    Supportive Oncology
Cleveland Clinic
Cleveland, OH

Pedro Pérez-Cruz, MD, MPH
Assistant Professor
Departamento Medicina Interna
Facultad de Medicina
Pontificia Universidad Católica
    de Chile
Santiago, Chile

**Peter Poon, MBBS, PGDipPM,
FRACGP, FAChPM**
Associate Professor and Director
Supportive and Palliative Care Unit
Monash Health
Melbourne, Australia

Eric Prommer, MD
University of California, Los Angeles/
    Veterans Affairs Hospice
    and Palliative Care
Associate Professor of Medicine
University of California, Los Angeles
    School of Medicine
Los Angeles, CA

**Bianca Sakamoto Ribeiro Paiva,
RN, PhD**
Professor Postgraduation program,
    Palliative Care and Quality of Life
    Research Group
Barretos Cancer Hospital
Barretos, Sao Paulo, Brazil

Alfredo Rodríguez-Núñez, MD
Programa Medicina Paliativa y
  Cuidados Continuos
Departamento Medicina Familiar
Facultad de Medicina
Pontificia Universidad Católica
  de Chile
Santiago, Chile

Eric J. Roeland, MD
Assistant Clinical Professor
Department of Oncology
University of California, San Diego
San Diego, CA

**Fiona Runacres, MBBS, (Hons),
FRACGP, FAChPM**
Palliative Care Specialist and Adjunct
  Clinical Lecturer
Supportive and Palliative Care Unit,
  Monash Health, Melbourne,
  Australia and Calvary Health Care
  Bethlehem
Melbourne, Australia

Yael Schenker, MD, MAS
Associate Professor of Medicine
Director, Palliative Care Research
Section of Palliative Care and Medical
  Ethics
Division of General Internal Medicine
University of Pittsburgh
Pittsburgh, PA

Tiffany Shaw, MD
Fellow, Hospice and Palliative
  Medicine
University of California, Los Angeles/
  Veterans Affairs Hospice and
  Palliative Care
Los Angeles, CA

Christian T. Sinclair, MD, FAAHPM
Assistant Professor, Division of
  Palliative Medicine
University of Kansas Health System
Kansas City, KS

Jesse A. Soodalter, MD, MA
Post-doctoral Research Fellow,
  Section of Palliative Care and
  Medical Ethics
University of Pittsburgh
Clinical Instructor, Palliative and
  Supportive Institute
University of Pittsburgh Medical
  Center Health System
Pittsburgh, PA

Kimberson Tanco, MD
Assistant Professor
Department of Palliative,
  Rehabilitation, and Integrative
  Medicine
Division of Cancer Medicine
The University of Texas MD
  Anderson Cancer Center
Houston, TX

Anna Cecilia Tenorio, MD
Fellow, Hospice and Palliative
  Medicine
Department of Palliative,
  Rehabilitation, and Integrative
  Medicine
The University of Texas MD
  Anderson Cancer Center
Division of Cancer Medicine
Houston, TX

Jason A. Webb, MD, FAPA
Director of Education, Duke Palliative
  Care
Program Director, Hospice and
  Palliative Medicine Fellowship
  Program
Assistant Professor, Department of
  Medicine
Assistant Professor, Department of
  Psychiatry and Behavioral Sciences
Duke University & Medical Center
Durham, NC

Eric Widera, MD
Professor of Clinical Medicine,
  Division of Geriatrics, University of
  California San Francisco (UCSF)
Program Director, Geriatric Medicine
  Fellowship, UCSF
Director, Hospice and Palliative Care,
  San Francisco Veterans Affairs
  Medical Center
San Francisco, CA

**Jaclyn Yoong, MBBS (Hons),
FRACP, FAChPM, MPH**
Medical Oncologist and Palliative
  Care Physician
Monash Health
Northern Health
Melbourne, Australia

Justin Yu, MD
Clinical Instructor of Medicine
Division of General Internal Medicine
  and Section of Palliative Care and
  Medical Ethics
University of Pittsburgh Medical
  Center
Pittsburgh, PA

**Donna S. Zhukovsky, MD,
FACP, FAAHPM**
Professor
Department of Palliative,
  Rehabilitation and Integrative
  Medicine
The University of Texas MD
  Anderson Cancer Center
Houston, TX

50 Studies Every Palliative Care Doctor Should Know

SECTION 1

Palliative Care

1

Early Palliative Care for Patients with Metastatic Non-Small Cell Lung Cancer

NATHAN A. GRAY AND THOMAS W. LEBLANC

> Early integration of palliative care for patients with non-small cell lung cancer . . . has effects on survival and quality of life that are similar to the effects of first-line chemotherapy in such patients.
>
> —Temel et al.[1]

Research Question: Does combining early palliative care with standard oncologic care improve patient-reported outcomes, use of health services, and quality of end-of-life care among patients with metastatic non-small cell lung cancer (NSCLC)?

Funding: American Society of Clinical Oncology (Career Development Award) and philanthropic gifts from Joanne Hill Monahan Cancer Fund and Golf Fights Cancer.

Year Study Began: 2006.

Year Study Published: 2010.

Study Location: Massachusetts General Hospital, Boston, MA.

Who Was Studied: Outpatients with pathologically confirmed metastatic NSCLC diagnosed within the prior 8 weeks and with Eastern Cooperative Oncology Group (ECOG) scale scores of ≤2.

Who Was Excluded: Patients who were already receiving palliative care services and those who were non-English speaking.

How Many Patients: 151.

Study Overview: This was a randomized trial of early palliative care in conjunction with standard oncologic care versus standard oncologic care alone in patients with recently diagnosed metastatic NSCLC. One hundred fifty-one patients were randomized on a 1:1 ratio. Patients in the standard oncologic care arm could still receive palliative care services if their oncologist, the patient, or family members requested them (Figure 1.1).

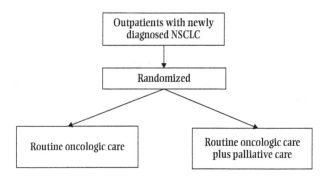

Figure 1.1 Summary of study design.

Study Intervention: Patients randomized to the intervention arm had a visit with one of the members of the palliative care team within 3 weeks of enrollment and at least monthly thereafter, with additional visits at the discretion of the patient, palliative care team, or oncologist. Palliative care visits generally followed the National Consensus Project for Quality Palliative Care guidelines, paying specific attention to treating physical and psychosocial symptoms, establishing goals of care, and coordinating care based on patient needs. Patients who were not assigned to the palliative care group were not referred to palliative care unless specifically requested by the patient, family, or oncologist. All participants received routine oncologic care throughout the study duration, at the discretion of the treating oncologist.

Follow-up: Assessments were performed at 12 weeks from date of enrollment.

Endpoints: The primary outcome was change in quality of life (QoL) at 12 weeks using the Trial Outcome Index (TOI) of the Functional Assessment of Cancer Therapy–Lung (FACT-L) scale (the TOI is the sum of the Lung Cancer subscale and the Physical Well-Being and Functional Well-Being subscales of the FACT-L instrument). Secondary outcomes included overall QoL, mood, health care utilization, and documentation of resuscitation preferences. QoL was assessed by the FACT-G scale and its Lung Cancer subscale, which together make up the FACT-L instrument. Mood was assessed using the Hospital Anxiety and Depression Scale and the Patient Health Questionnaire–9. At death, data were collected from the electronic medical record regarding the use of health services and end-of-life care. These data included prescriptions, anti-cancer therapy use, hospice referrals, hospital admissions, and date/location of death. Patients were classified as having received "aggressive care" if they had any of the following outcomes: chemotherapy within 14 days of death, no use of hospice care, or admission to hospice ≤3 days before death. Survival was measured in days from time of enrollment.

RESULTS

- In general, the early palliative care group had improved QoL, fewer depressive symptoms, and longer overall (median) survival (Table 1.1).

Table 1.1. SUMMARY OF STUDY'S KEY FINDINGS

	Standard Care	Early Palliative Care	Difference Between Groups (95% CI)	P Value
TOI	53.0±11.5	59.0±11.6	6.0 (1.5–10.4)	0.009
FACT-L score (quality of life)	91.5±15.8	98.0±15.1	6.5 (0.5–12.4)	0.03
Depressive symptoms	38%	16%	—	0.01
Aggressive end-of-life care	54%	33%	—	0.05
Median survival (months)	8.9	11.6	—	0.02

NOTE: CI = confidence interval; TOI = Trial Outcome Index; FACT-L = Functional Assessment of Cancer Therapy–Lung.

- The primary outcome, the TOI of the FACT-L instrument, showed significant improvements at 12 weeks for those in the early palliative care group (the mean change in TOI was positive for the early palliative care arm and negative for the standard care arm).
- Overall QoL by the FACT-L was also significantly better in the early palliative care group.
- Patients in the early palliative care arm reported fewer depressive symptoms at 12 weeks.
- Despite receiving less aggressive end-of-life care according to the composite secondary endpoint, patients in the palliative care group demonstrated longer median survival by approximately 2.5 months.

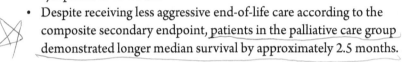

Criticisms and Limitations:

- The study was performed at a single, tertiary care site with a high level of specialty palliative care and oncology support in a population that lacked diversity.
- Study was not blinded; patients and treating providers were aware of assignment.
- Patients receiving the palliative care intervention received additional clinical visits, as there were no control visits for the standard care arm, raising the possibility that benefits were a manifestation of closer clinical supervision.

Other Relevant Studies and Information:

- Subsequent studies by Temel and colleagues have further characterized the nature and scope of their palliative care intervention visits as well as attempted to determine which patient subsets might benefit most from palliative care involvement.[2,3] However, the means by which palliative care influenced survival outcomes remains poorly understood.
- The ENABLE trial in 2013 demonstrated improvement in survival for patients receiving early versus delayed initiation of palliative care in a broader population of cancer patients but did not demonstrate statistically different changes in resource utilization or QoL.[4] Similarly, a large cluster-randomized trial by Zimmermann et al. demonstrated improvements in symptoms and QoL but not survival with early concurrent palliative care in a broader population of patients with advanced solid tumors.[5]

- Early palliative care has been suggested as potentially beneficial for patients suffering from many other illnesses, including heart failure and neurodegenerative disorders, but additional evidence is needed.[6–8]
- Since 2010, developments in antineoplastic options, including immunotherapy and expansion in novel targeted therapies, have transformed the landscape of prognosis and toxicity for patients with NSCLC and indeed cancer in general. While the principles of meticulous symptom assessment, psychosocial support, and clear communication are presumably still beneficial to patients, the impact of specialty palliative care has not yet been rigorously studied in this newer, more complex environment.[9] Such studies are ongoing.
- A follow-up study by Temel et al. compared early palliative care to usual oncology care for patients with lung and gastrointestinal malignancies. This study found that QoL and mood improved from baseline to week 24 (secondary outcome) but not at week 12 (primary outcome). Early benefit was observed more among patients with lung cancer than gastrointestinal cancer.[10]

Summary and Implications: This landmark randomized trial of early palliative care among patients with metastatic NSCLC demonstrated that patients who were referred at the time of diagnosis benefitted from improved QoL, decreased rates of depression, decreased use of aggressive care at the end of life, and improved survival.

CLINICAL CASE: WHO SHOULD BE REFERRED TO PALLIATIVE CARE?

Case History

A 58-year-old woman with metastatic adenocarcinoma of the lung is seen in oncology clinic for her first visit following a recent diagnosis of lung cancer. She initially presented to her primary care provider for cough and weight loss, and she otherwise appears relatively asymptomatic. She has an ECOG performance status of 1. Her oncologist plans to start first-line palliative-intent chemotherapy but wonders if there is any reason to refer to palliative care now, rather than waiting until symptoms worsen or until there are no remaining options to treat her cancer.

Is it too early to refer to palliative care?

Suggested Answer

The trial by Temel and colleagues introduced palliative care to patients with metastatic NSCLC with good performance near the time of initial diagnosis, rather than waiting for symptom- or crisis-driven referral.

The patient presented in this case matches the eligibility profile of patients in the study, and the study results suggest that she could benefit from lower rates of depression, improved QoL, and potentially improved survival. Additionally, early referral may simultaneously decrease her likelihood of receiving aggressive care interventions such as chemotherapy at the end of her life, which would not be consistent with many patients' goals. Although her primary oncologist may provide symptom-directed care and continuing discussions of goals (i.e., "primary palliative care"), it appears that the addition of a dedicated team of specialist-trained palliative providers may confer further advantages in addressing her needs beyond the primary palliative care provided by the cancer care team.

Thus, while planning for initial cancer-directed therapy, the oncologist should suggest that the patient consider visiting concurrently with a palliative care clinician and make a referral if the patient is interested.

References

1. Temel JS, Greer JA, Muzikansky A, et al. Early palliative care for patients with metastatic non–small-cell lung cancer. *N Engl J Med.* 2010;363(8):733–742.
2. Jacobsen J, Jackson V, Dahlin C, et al. Components of early outpatient palliative care consultation in patients with metastatic nonsmall cell lung cancer. *J Palliat Med.* 2011;14(4):459–464.
3. Nipp RD, Greer JA, El-Jawahri A, et al. Age and gender moderate the impact of early palliative care in metastatic non-small cell lung cancer. *Oncologist.* 2016;21(1):119–126.
4. Bakitas MA, Tosteson TD, Li Z, et al. Early versus delayed initiation of concurrent palliative oncology care: patient outcomes in the ENABLE III randomized controlled trial. *J Clin Oncol.* 2015;33(13):1438-45.
5. Zimmermann C, Swami N, Krzyzanowska M, et al. Early palliative care for patients with advanced cancer: a cluster-randomised controlled trial. *Lancet.* 2014;383(9930):1721–1730.
6. Higginson IJ, Costantini M, Silber E, Burman R, Edmonds P. Evaluation of a new model of short-term palliative care for people severely affected with multiple sclerosis: a randomised fast-track trial to test timing of referral and how long the effect is maintained. *Postgrad Med J.* 2011;87(1033):769–775.
7. Parikh RB, Kirch RA, Smith TJ, Temel JS. Early specialty palliative care—translating data in oncology into practice. *N Engl J Med.* 2013;369(24):2347–2351.

8. Hauptman PJ, Havranek EP. Integrating palliative care into heart failure care. *Arch Intern Med.* 2005;165(4):374–378.

9. Temel JS, Shaw AT, Greer JA. Challenge of prognostic uncertainty in the modern era of cancer therapeutics. *J Clin Oncol.* 2016;34(30):3605–3608.

10. Temel JS, Greer JA, El-Jawahri A, et al. Effects of early integrated palliative care in patients with lung and GI cancer: a randomized clinical trial. *J Clin Oncol.* 2017;35(8):834—841.

2

Early Palliative Care for Patients with Advanced Cancer

DAVID HUI

> This trial shows promising findings that support early palliative care for patients with advanced cancer.
>
> —ZIMMERMANN ET AL.[1]

Research Question: Does early introduction of palliative care improve quality of life, symptom burden, patient satisfaction, and communication in patients with advanced cancer?

Funding: Canadian Cancer Society, Ontario Ministry of Health and Long Term Care.

Year Study Began: 2006.

Year Study Published: 2014.

Study Location: Princess Margaret Cancer Centre, Toronto, Canada.

Who Was Studied: Adults with advanced solid tumors (lung, gastrointestinal, genitourinary, breast, and gynecological) with a prognosis of 6 to 24 months and an Eastern Cooperative Oncology Group performance of 0 to 2.

Who Was Excluded: Patients with insufficient English literacy.

How Many Patients: 461.

Study Overview: This is a cluster randomized controlled trial in which 24 oncologists were randomized to either early palliative care or usual care in a 1:1 ratio, stratified by clinic size and tumor type. Patients in both groups received routine oncologic care. This design allows for partial blinding because patients only consented to participate in the assigned arm and were not made aware of the other study arm (Figure 2.1).

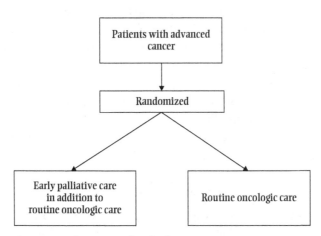

Figure 2.1 Summary of study design.

Study Intervention: Patients in the early palliative care group received an outpatient consultation by the palliative care team (a physician and nurse for 60–90 minutes) within 1 month of recruitment, a brief telephone follow-up call 1 week after the consultation, and were followed by monthly clinic visits (20–50 minutes each). During each visit, the patients completed structured assessments of their physical and psychosocial distress and received interdisciplinary care addressing their physical, emotional, social, and spiritual needs. Patients also had access to the palliative care inpatient consultation service and home care service if needed. They also received routine care from their oncologists.

Patients in the control group received usual oncologic care. Although they would not be automatically referred to palliative care, the attending oncologists had the option to refer patients to palliative care as per routine practice. Only 9% of these control patients had an outpatient palliative care clinic visit.

Follow-up: 4 months.

Endpoints: Primary outcome: Quality of life (Functional Assessment of Chronic Illness Therapy–Spiritual Well-Being [FACIT-Sp]) at 3 months. Secondary outcomes: Quality of life (FACIT-Sp at 4 months, Quality of Life at the End-of-Life [QUAL-E]) at 3 and 4 months; symptom burden (Edmonton Symptom Assessment Scale [ESAS]), patient satisfaction (FAMCARE-P16), patient-clinician communication (Cancer Rehabilitation Evaluation System Medical Interaction Subscale [CARES-MIS]) at 3 and 4 months.

RESULTS

- In general, the early palliative care group had improved quality of life, symptom burden, and patient satisfaction over the 4-month study period. In contrast, the control group had worsened outcomes over time.
- The primary outcome (FACIT-Sp at 3 months) was better in the palliative care arm, albeit not statistically significant. It became significant at 4 months (Table 2.1).
- The secondary outcomes QUAL-E, ESAS, and FAMCARE-P16 all favored the palliative care group (Table 2.1).

Table 2.1. SUMMARY OF STUDY'S KEY FINDINGS

	Palliative Care 3 Months	Oncologic Care 3 Months	P Value	Palliative Care 4 Months	Oncologic Care 4 Months	P Value
FACIT-Sp	1.6±14.5	−2.0±13.6	0.07	2.5±15.5	−4.0±14.2	0.006
QUAL-E	2.3 (8.3)	0.06 (8.3)	0.05	3.0 (8.3)	−0.51 (7.6)	0.003
ESAS	0.1±16.9	2.1±13.9	0.33	−1.3±16.0	3.2±13.9	0.05
FAMCARE-P16	2.3±9.1	−1.8±8.2	0.0003	3.7±8.6	−2.4±8.3	< 0.0001
CARES-MIS	−0.2 (5.5)	0.9 (4.1)	0.02	-0.4 (4.4)	0.6 (3.6)	0.02

NOTE: FACIT-Sp = Functional Assessment of Chronic Illness Therapy–Spiritual Well-Being; QUAL-E = Quality of Life at the End-of-Life; ESAS = Edmonton Symptom Assessment Scale; CARES-MIS = Cancer Rehabilitation Evaluation System Medical Interaction Subscale.

Criticisms and Limitations:

- Strictly speaking, this could be termed a negative trial because the primary outcome did not reach statistical significance. However, from a pragmatic standpoint, the outcomes all favored the palliative care arm compared to the control arm. Overall, this study provides convincing evidence to support early involvement of palliative care for patients with advanced cancer.

- This is a single-center study with a comprehensive palliative care team in a large tertiary care cancer center. It is unclear if the findings are generalizable to other settings.
- Research staff conducting the study assessments and the palliative care team delivering the study intervention were not blinded to the assignment, which may potentially contribute to bias given that the study outcomes were subjective in nature.

Other Relevant Studies and Information:

- Compared to the Temel trial (see chapter 1),[2] this study was larger, included patients with multiple types of advanced solid tumors, incorporated a cluster randomization design that allowed for partial blinding, used prognosis instead of time from diagnosis to trigger referral, and examined different outcomes. Survival could not be examined because prognosis was one of the eligibility criteria.
- The outpatient clinic was described in further detail in a subsequent article.[3]
- The investigators also conducted a qualitative study to examine the roles perceived by patients enrolled into this trial of their palliative care and oncology teams. Patients in the intervention group reported that the care received by the palliative care team offered a distinct and complementary approach to their oncologists.[4]
- Following evidence from this and other studies, the 2017 American Society of Clinical Oncology Clinical Practice Guideline recommends that patients with advanced cancer should receive dedicated palliative care services early in the disease course, concurrent with active treatment.[5]

Summary and Implications: This large cluster randomized controlled trial demonstrated improved quality of life, symptom burden, and satisfaction among patients with advanced cancer who were referred for early palliative care versus. controls who were not immediately referred. It is the largest study to date on this topic and the only one of this kind to incorporate a partially blinded approach to minimize bias.

CLINICAL CASE: WHO SHOULD BE REFERRED TO PALLIATIVE CARE?

Case History

A 65-year-old man with newly diagnosed stage IV renal cell cancer is about to start first-line treatment with pazopanib. He has mild right flank pain and no weight loss. He has a performance status of 1. His oncologist told him that his prognosis is approximately 1 year. He is anxious about his cancer diagnosis but has no clinical depression.

Should this patient be referred to palliative care?

Suggested Answer

The Zimmermann trial introduced palliative care to patients with advanced cancer who had a good performance status and a prognosis of 6 to 24 months, regardless of symptom burden, and found that there was improvement in quality of life, symptom burden, and patient satisfaction over time.

The patient in this case scenario would meet the eligibility criteria and would benefit from a referral to palliative care. Although our patient appears to have a low symptom burden at this time, palliative care may detect unmet physical and emotional needs, and he is likely to experience a greater number of symptoms as his disease progresses. While the oncologist can provide primary palliative care directly, randomized controlled trials clearly demonstrate that the *addition* of palliative care to oncologic care is associated with improved patient outcomes. Furthermore, early involvement of the interprofessional palliative care team may enhance psychosocial support, improve illness understanding, and facilitate care planning.

Thus the oncologist may want to start a conversation with the patient about the benefits of concurrent palliative care and make a referral if the patient is interested.

References

1. Zimmermann C, Swami N, Krzyzanowska M, et al. Early palliative care for patients with advanced cancer: a cluster-randomised controlled trial. *Lancet.* 2014 May 17;383(9930):1721–1730.
2. Temel JS, Greer JA, Muzikansky A, et al. Early palliative care for patients with metastatic non-small-cell lung cancer. *N Engl J Med.* 2010 Aug 19;363(8):733–742.
3. Hannon B, Swami N, Pope A, et al. The oncology palliative care clinic at the Princess Margaret Cancer Centre: an early intervention model for patients with advanced cancer. *Support Care Cancer.* 2015 Apr;23(4):1073–1080.

4. Hannon B, Swami N, Pope A, et al. Early palliative care and its role in oncology: a qualitative study. *Oncologist.* 2016 Jul 22. pii: theoncologist.2016–0176
5. Ferrell BR, Temel JS, Temin S, et al. Integration of palliative care into standard oncology care: American Society of Clinical Oncology Clinical Practice Guideline update. *J Clin Oncol.* 2017 Jan;35(1):96–112

3

Nurse-Led Palliative Care for Advanced Cancer Patients

EMILY J. MARTIN AND ERIC J. ROELAND

> This is the first randomized controlled trial designed to test a palliative care intervention concurrent with oncology treatment.
>
> —BAKITAS ET AL.[1]

Research Question: How does a nurse-led palliative care intervention impact quality of life, symptom intensity, mood, and resource use among advanced cancer patients?

Funding: National Cancer Institute grant.

Year Study Began: 2003.

Year Study Published: 2009.

Study Location: Norris Cotton Cancer Center and affiliated outreach clinics in New Hampshire and a VA medical center in Vermont.

Who Was Studied: Patients who received a new diagnosis of advanced cancer with a life expectancy of approximately 1 year within 8 to 12 weeks prior to enrolment. These patients were identified during tumor board meetings. Advanced cancer diagnoses included unresectable stage III or IV gastrointestinal cancer; stage IIIB or IV non-small cell or extensive small cell lung cancer; stage IV genitourinary cancer; or stage IV breast cancer (with visceral crisis, lung or liver metastases, ER negative, Her 2/neu positive).

Who Was Excluded: Patients with impaired cognition (score <17 on the modified Mini-Mental State Examination), schizophrenia or bipolar disorder, or active substance use.

How Many Patients: 322 (161 in each arm).

Study Overview: This randomized controlled trial examined the effect of a palliative care intervention compared to usual oncologic care on quality of life, symptom intensity, resource use, and mood among patients recently diagnosed with new, recurrent, or progressive cancer (with an estimated life expectancy of 1 year). Patients were randomly assigned 1:1 to either the control (usual care) group or the palliative care intervention group using a stratified block system (stratified based on disease and site). Patients completed a baseline questionnaire at time of enrolment as well as a questionnaire at 1 month and subsequently every 3 months until study completion or patient's death (Figure 3.1).

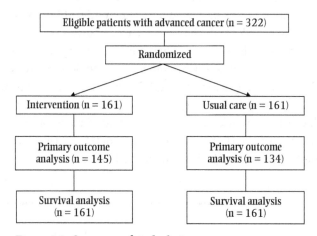

Figure 3.1 Summary of study design.

Study Intervention: ENABLE ("Educate, Nurture, Advise Before Life Ends") is a nurse-led, psychoeducational, case-management model based on the chronic care model completed between 2003 and 2008.[2] The intervention was started following enrollment, randomization, and baseline assessment. It included four educational telephone sessions, led by one of two advanced practice nurses followed by at least monthly telephone calls until the time of the patient's death for continued assessment of new or ongoing issues. The advanced practice nurses had undergone 20 hours of specialized palliative care training prior to the study. The four structured telephone sessions, using the "Charting Your Course: An Intervention for People and Families Living with Cancer" guidebook, addressed problem-solving, symptom management, communication/social support, and advance care planning. The sessions averaged 30 to 40 minutes each. Patients in the intervention group were also invited to participate in monthly group-shared medical appointments, which provided an opportunity to address medical issues that required more time than was feasible during a routine clinic visit.

Patients assigned to the usual care group were permitted to use all available supportive services (including referral to palliative care).

Follow-up: Questionnaires every 3 months until patient's death or study completion.

Endpoints: Primary outcomes included quality of life, symptom intensity, and resource use. Mood was a secondary outcome. Quality of life was measured by the Functional Assessment of Chronic Illness Therapy–Palliative Care (FACIT-Pal),[3] which uses a scale of 0 to 184 with higher scores indicating greater quality of life. Symptom intensity was measured using the modified Edmonton Symptom Assessment Scale (ESAS),[4] which uses a scale of 0 to 10 to assess symptoms of pain, activity, nausea, depression, anxiety, drowsiness, appetite, sense of well-being, and shortness of breath with higher scores indicating greater symptom intensity. Resource use (including length of hospital stay, length of intensive care unit [ICU] stay, and number of emergency department visits) was evaluating through chart review. Mood was assessed by the Center for Epidemiological Studies Depression Scale (CES-D)[5] with a scale of 0 to 60 (with scores of 16 or greater indicating clinically significant depressed mood).

RESULTS

- A total of 1,222 patients were screened. Of these, 681 were eligible and 322 enrolled (participation rate of 47%); these patients were randomly assigned to either the control group (usual care) or the intervention group (161 patients assigned to each group).

- 27 patients in the usual care group and 16 patients in the intervention group withdrew or died, leaving 134 patients in the usual care group and 145 in the intervention group for analysis of patient-reported outcomes. Reasons for withdrawal were not detailed.
- There were no statistically significant differences between the two groups in baseline demographic characteristics, clinical characteristics, quality of life, symptom intensity, or depressed mood.
- Longitudinal intention-to-treat analyses showed statistically significant higher quality of life (P = 0.02) and less depressed mood (P = 0.02) as well as a trend toward lower symptom intensity (P = 0.06) in the intervention group (Table 3.1).

Table 3.1. Summary of Study's Key Findings—Longitudinal Intention-to-Treat Analysis: Palliative Care Intervention Plus Usual Oncologic Care Compared to Usual Oncologic Care

	Mean (Standard Error)	P Value
QoL (FACIT-PAL)	4.6 (2)	0.02
Symptom Intensity (ESAS)	−27.8 (15)	0.06
Depressed Mood (CES-D)	−1.8 (0.81)	0.02

NOTE: QoL = quality of life; FACIT-PAL = Functional Assessment of Chronic Illness Therapy–Palliative Care; ESAS = Edmonton Symptom Assessment Scale; CES-D = Center for Epidemiological Studies Depression Scale.

- Improved quality of life and mood in the intervention group were both statistically and clinically significant (based on the FACIT-Pal tool and using a distribution-based approach).
- There were no statistically significant differences in the number of patients who received chemotherapy (P = 0.80) or radiation therapy (P = 0.89) between the two groups.
- There were no statistically significant differences in median survival (intervention group 14 months [95% confidence interval (CI), 10.6–18.4 months] and 8.5 months [95% CI, 7.0–11.1 months]) for the usual care group (P = 0.14) or resource use (days in hospital [P = 0.14], days in ICU [P > 0.99], or number of emergency department visits [P = 0.53]) between the two groups (Table 3.2).
- There was no statistically significant difference in symptom intensity (based on ESAS) between groups.

Table 3.2. SUMMARY OF STUDY'S KEY FINDINGS—RESOURCE USE

	Intervention Group	Control Group	P Value
Hospital Days	6.6	6.5	0.14
ICU Days	0.06	0.06	>0.99
Emergency Department Visits	0.86	0.63	0.53

NOTE: ICU = intensive care unit.

Criticisms and Limitations:

- Limited ethnic and racial diversity in the patient population make it unclear how generalizable the results are to the larger population.
- The intervention was largely limited to telephone, nurse-led encounters (i.e., an advanced practice nurse was the key entry point to the provision of palliative care), which may not be as effective as in-person, longitudinal, interdisciplinary palliative care clinic visits. This model of care may be particularly appropriate for rural and resource-scare settings.
- Chart review may not have fully captured resource use.
- Inclusion of a wide variety of cancer types may have resulted in a heterogeneous sample population resulting in decreased signal.
- The lack of difference in end-of-life resource use may be explained partly by floor effect.

Other Relevant Studies and Information:

- The palliative care intervention used in this study used the "Charting Your Course: An Intervention for People and Families Living with Cancer" curriculum initially developed in Project ENABLE demonstration project.[6]
- Building upon the results of this study, Project ENABLE III examined the effect of early versus delayed palliative care intervention in patients with advanced cancer.[7]
- Since the publication of this study, several organizations including the American Society of Clinical Oncology and the National Comprehensive Cancer Network have released clinical guidelines recommending the incorporation of palliative care into the management of oncologic care at the time of diagnosis of advanced-stage cancer.[8,9]
- Project ENABLE II is the only palliative care intervention recommended by the National Cancer Institute Research Tested Intervention Program as being ready for dissemination into practice.

Summary and Implications: This study showed that the addition of a telephone-based, nurse-led palliative care intervention to usual oncologic care was associated with higher quality of life and less depressed mood compared to usual care alone. While there was a trend toward decreased symptom intensity and increased survival in the intervention group, these associations did not reach statistical significance. There was no significant difference in resource use between the two groups.

CLINICAL CASE: WHO SHOULD BE REFERRED TO PALLIATIVE CARE?

Case History

A 58-year-old man with recently diagnosed stage IIIB non-small cell lung cancer returns to the cancer clinic to further discuss initiation of chemotherapy. He is feeling well, with no specific symptoms at this time. He lives 2 hours from the hospital and states he is concerned about his ability to make it to his appointments were his health to decline. His oncologist informs him that his life expectancy is approximately 12 months.

Should this patient be referred to palliative care?

Suggested Answer

Project ENABLE II demonstrated improved quality of life and less depressed mood in patients who received a telephone-based, nurse-led palliative care intervention in conjunction with usual oncologic care. The study also showed a trend toward decreased symptom intensity and increased survival in those that received the palliative care intervention.

This patient would likely benefit from a referral to palliative care. Based on the findings in Project ENABLE II and given the patient's distance from the hospital, a telephone-based intervention addressing problem-solving, communication and social support, symptom management, and advance care planning may be particularly beneficial in this patient's case. While this patient denies acute symptoms at this time, palliative care would be able to address his symptoms if and when they arise as a result of chemotherapy and/or disease progression.

References

1. Bakitas M, Lyons K, Hegel M, et al. Effects of a palliative care intervention on clinical outcomes in patients with advanced cancer: the Project ENABLE II randomized controlled trial. *JAMA.* 2009;302(7):741–749.

2. Bakitas M, Lyons K, Hegel M, et al. Project ENABLE II randomized controlled trial to improve palliative care for rural patients with advanced cancer: baseline findings, methodological challenges, and solutions. *Palliat Support Care.* 2009;7(1):75–86.
3. Lyons KD, Bakitas M, Hegel MT, et al. Reliability and validity of the Functional Assessment of Chronic Illness Therapy–Palliative Care (FACIT-Pal) scale. *J Pain Symptom Manage.* 2009;37(1):23–32.
4. Bruera E, Kuehn N, Miller MJ et al. The Edmonton Symptom Assessment System (ESAS): a simple method for the assessment of palliative care patients. *J Palliat Care.* 1991;7(2):6–9.
5. Radloff L. The CES-D Scale: a self-report depression scale for research in the general population. *Appl Psychol Meas.* 1977;1:385–401.
6. Bakitas M, Stevens M, Ahles T, et al. Project ENABLE: a palliative care demonstration project for advanced cancer patients in three settings. *J Palliat Med.* 2004; 7(2):363–372.
7. Bakitas M, Tosteson TD, Li Z, et al. Early versus delayed initiation of concurrent palliative oncology care: patient outcomes in the ENABLE III randomized controlled trial. *J Clin Oncol.* 2015;33(13):1438–1445.
8. Ferrell BR, Temel JS, Temin S, et al. Integration of palliative care into standard oncology care: American Society of Clinical Oncology Clinical Practice Guideline update. *J Clin Oncol.* 2017;35(1):96–112.
9. National Comprehensive Cancer Network. *NCCN clinical practice guidelines in oncology: palliative care.* Retrieved from http://www.nccn.org/professionals/physician_gls/f_guidelines.asp

4

Benefits of Early Palliative Care to Informal Family Caregivers

EMILY J. MARTIN AND ERIC J. ROELAND

> This was the first early intervention trial to our knowledge that provided a specific intervention for [caregivers].
>
> —DIONNE-ODOM ET AL.[1]

Research Question: Does early versus delayed palliative care intervention for family caregivers impact caregiver quality of life, depression scores, or stress/demand/objective burden?

Funding: National Institutes for Nursing Research, National Cancer Institute, National Institutes of Health's National Institute of Nursing Research Small Research Grant, and Mentored Research Scholar Grant in Applied and Clinical Research from the American Cancer Society.

Year Study Began: 2010.

Year Study Published: 2013.

Study Location: Norris Cotton Cancer Center, affiliated outreach clinics, and the VA Medical Center in New Hampshire and Vermont.

Who Was Studied: Primary caregivers of patients with advanced stage cancer (new diagnosis, recurrence, or progression within 30–60 days) with a prognosis of 6 to 24 months. Caregivers were defined as "a person who knows you well and is involved in your medical care."[1]

Who Was Excluded: No formal caregiver exclusion criteria.

How Many Patients: 122 caregivers.

Study Overview: This is a randomized controlled trial with a fast-track design where all caregivers received the intervention but those assigned to the early (fast-track) group received the intervention soon after the time of assignment while caregivers in the delayed group received the intervention 3 months after assignment (Figure 4.1).

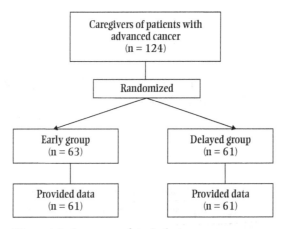

Figure 4.1 Summary of study design.

Study Intervention: Three weekly one-on-one telephone sessions between one of seven advanced practice palliative care nurses (who had received approximately 30 hours of training) and a caregiver. The telephone sessions were structured based on the "Charting Your Course: Caregiver" guidebook. Session 1 focused on the process of adopting the caregiver role, understanding the role of palliative and supportive care, and outlining problem-solving skills. Session 2 addressed caregiver self-care as well as patient symptom assessment and management. Session 3 covered utilizing a support team, decision-making, decision support, and advance care planning. The sessions averaged 23 minutes in duration.

The 3 weekly sessions were followed by at least monthly telephone calls from the advanced practice palliative care nurse to address new or ongoing issues until the patient's death or the end of the study.

The early group received this intervention just after random assignment. The delayed group received the intervention 3 months after random assignment.

Follow-up: Telephone-based questionnaires were administered every 6 weeks until week 24 and then every 3 months until the patient's death or completion of the study.

Endpoints: Primary outcomes included caregiver quality of life as assessed by the Caregiver Quality of Life Scale–Cancer (CQOL-C), depression as assessed by the Center for Epidemiologic Study-Depression (CESD) Scale, and burden as assessed by the Montgomery-Borgatta Caregiver Burden (MBCB) Scale with subscales for objective, demand, and stress burden.

RESULTS

- Of the 124 identified caregivers, 122 enrolled in the study.
- There were no significant differences in baseline characteristics between caregivers in the early and delayed groups except there were more employed caregivers in the early group, $P = 0.05$ (Tables 4.1 and 4.2).
- There were no significant differences in the outcome measures between the early and delayed groups at baseline.
- The majority of caregivers (75%) were the patient's partner or spouse.
- Most of the caregivers cared for a patient with lung (43%) or gastrointestinal (25%) cancer.
- 32% of caregivers did not complete all follow-up evaluations.
- At 3 months, caregivers in early group had a significantly improved depression score from baseline compared to caregivers in the delayed group ($P = 0.02$).
- There were no significant differences in quality of life or burden between the early and delayed groups.
- Terminal decline analysis of caregivers of patients that died during the study showed significant between group differences favoring the early group for depression and stress burden but not for quality of life, objective burden, or demand burden.
- In the 3 months before death, the average depression scores for caregivers in the delayed group met criteria for clinically significant depression.

Table 4.1. SUMMARY OF STUDY'S KEY FINDINGS—ENDPOINTS AT BASELINE,
1.5 MONTHS, AND 3 MONTHS

Assessment	Month After Baseline	Early Group No. Caregivers	Mean Score (SE)	Delayed Group No. Caregivers	Mean Score (SE)
Quality of Life (CQOL-C)					
	0	61	58.5 (2.0)	61	62.4 (2.0)
	1.5	39	52.2 (2.3)	44	58.0 (2.2)
	3	35	50.2 (2.4)	34	55.7 (2.4)
Depression (CESD)					
	0	60	13.4 (1.3)	58	15.9 (1.4)
	1.5	39	8.8 (1.5)	44	15.9 (1.4)
	3	35	10.2 (1.5)	34	14.1 (1.6)
Objective Burden (MBCB-OB)					
	0	61	22.4 (0.5)	59	22.5 (0.5)
	1.5	39	22.1 (0.6)	44	21.7 (0.5)
	3	35	22.2 (0.6)	34	22.2 (0.6)
Stress Burden (MBCB-SB)					
	0	60	14.3 (0.3)	59	15.0 (0.3)
	1.5	38	13.2 (0.4)	44	14.3 (0.4)
	3	35	13.3 (0.4)	34	14.8 (0.4)
Demand Burden (MBCB-DB)					
	0	46	11.0 (0.5)	40	12.1 (0.5)
	1.5	30	10.6 (0.6)	34	11.6 (0.5)
	3	26	10.3 (0.6)	29	11.7 (0.6)

NOTE: SE = standard error; CESD = Center for Epidemiologic Studies–Depression Scale; CQOL-C = Caregiver Quality of Life Scale–Cancer; DB = demand burden; MBCB = Montgomery–Borgatta Caregiver Burden Scale; OB = objective burden; SB = stress burden.

Table 4.2. SUMMARY OF STUDY'S KEY FINDINGS—BETWEEN-GROUP DIFFERENCE
(EARLY MINUS DELAYED GROUP) IN CHANGE FROM BASELINE

Assessment	Mean	SE	P	Effect Size
Quality of Life (CQOL-C)	−2.1	2.3	0.37	−0.13
Depression (CESD)	−3.4	1.5	−0.32	−0.32
Objective Burden (MBCB-OB)	0.3	0.7	0.09	0.09
Stress Burden (MBCB-SB)	−0.6	0.5	−0.21	−0.21
Demand Burden (MBCB-DB)	0	0.7	0.99	0

NOTE: SE = standard error; CESD = Center for Epidemiologic Studies–Depression
Scale; CQOL-C = Caregiver Quality of Life Scale–Cancer; DB = demand burden;
MBCB = Montgomery–Borgatta Caregiver Burden Scale; OB = objective burden;
SB = stress burden.

Criticisms and Limitations:

- Small sample size due to low recruitment and high attrition.
- 32% of caregivers did not complete all of the follow-up assessments, which may have been due to increasing responsibilities associated with progressive patient illness (although, of note, there were no significant associations between outcomes or caregiver characteristics and attrition).
- Potential selection bias exists given the study did not meet the sample accrual goal.
- There are potential limits in generalizability (caregivers were predominantly Caucasian, female, at least high school educated, and located in a rural/small geographic area).

Other Relevant Studies and Information:

- The 2013 National Consensus Project for Quality Palliative Care recommends that palliative care efforts address both the needs of cancer patients and their caregivers.[2]
- A prior study, Project ENABLE II, demonstrated improved quality of life, depressed mood, and symptom intensity in advanced cancer patients who received early palliative care intervention.[3] These benefits

were not seen among the patients' caregivers, possibly due to lack of dedicated caregiver palliative care intervention.

- The parent study, Project ENABLE III, compared patient outcomes between early and delayed palliative care groups and revealed no difference in quality of life or mood. However, significant contamination in the control arm and suboptimal recruitment likely contributed to the negative findings.[1]
- The caregiver-specific palliative care intervention employed in this trial was designed to further assess the potential role of palliative care interventions for caregivers of patients with advanced cancer.[4]
- The 2015 study by Sun et al.[5] examining quality of life, psychological distress, burden, and caregiving skills preparedness among caregivers of patients with non-small cell lung cancer also demonstrated the benefits of caregiver-focused palliative care intervention; specifically, this study showed improved quality of life as well as lower psychological distress and objective burden in the group receiving the palliative care intervention.

Summary and Implications: This randomized controlled trial showed that caregivers of advanced cancer patients benefitted from earlier palliative care intervention. Specifically, caregivers who received palliative care intervention at the time of enrollment had lower depression scores at 3 months as well as lower depression and stress burden scores in the terminal decline analysis compared to caregivers who received palliative care intervention 3 months after time of enrollment. This study suggests that palliative care for caregivers of advanced cancer patients should be initiated as early as possible to improve caregiver depression and stress.

CLINICAL CASE: WHO SHOULD BE REFERRED TO PALLIATIVE CARE?

Case History

A 45-year-old woman presents to the oncology clinic with her husband to discuss her new diagnosis of stage IV breast cancer. She and her husband are struggling to process the prognosis of approximately 12 months. The patient is feeling well today but is afraid of suffering during her last months of life. Her husband asks what he can do to help his wife with any symptoms that arise. You decide to place a referral to palliative care for the patient. Should the patient's husband be referred to palliative care as well?

Suggested Answer

Caregivers of advanced cancer patients are at risk for depression, stress, and reduced quality of life. The Dionne-Odom trial suggests that caregivers of advanced cancer patients who received a telephone-based, nurse-led palliative care intervention soon after the time of diagnosis had lower depression and stress burden scores compared to caregivers who received the palliative care intervention 3 months after diagnosis. Based on this study, the patient's husband would likely benefit from a referral to palliative care. Such an intervention would be able to help him address the process of adopting the caregiver role, understanding palliative care, establishing a framework for problem-solving, maintaining self-care, assessing his wife's symptoms, utilizing available resources, and outlining advance care planning.

References

1. Dionne-Odom JN, Azuero A, Lyons KD, et al. Benefits of early versus delayed palliative care to informal family caregivers of patients with advanced cancer: outcomes from the ENABLE III randomized controlled trial. *J Clin Oncol*. 2015;33:1446–1452.
2. National Consensus Project for Quality Palliative Care. *clinical practice guidelines for quality palliative care*. 3rd ed. Pittsburgh, PA: National Consensus Project; 2013. Retrieved from www.nationalconsensusproject.org
3. Bakitas M, Lyons K, Hegel M, et al. Effects of a palliative care intervention on clinical outcomes in patients with advanced cancer: the Project ENABLE II randomized controlled trial. *JAMA*. 2009;302:741–749.
4. Williams AL, Bakitas M. Cancer family caregivers: a new direction for interventions. *J Palliat Med*. 2012;15:775–783.
5. Sun V, Grant M, Koczywas M, et al: Effectiveness of an interdisciplinary palliative care intervention for family caregivers in lung cancer. *Cancer*. 2015;121:3737–3745.

5

The Optimal Delivery of Palliative Care

JACLYN YOONG AND PETER POON

Care received in palliative care units may offer more improvements in care than those achieved with palliative care consultations.

—CASARETT ET AL.[1]

Research Question: Is the quality of [palliative] care provided by dedicated palliative care units better than that of palliative care consultation teams?

Funding/Support: Material based on work supported by the U.S. Department of Veterans Affairs (VA), Veterans Health Administration, Office of Research and Development, Human Services Research and Development. Funded as part of a grant from the Department of Veterans Affairs Comprehensive End-of-Life Care Initiative.

Year Study Began: 2008.

Year Study Published: 2011.

Study Location: 77 VA inpatient facilities in the United States and Puerto Rico with both palliative care consultation services and palliative care units.

Who Was Studied: Family members of patients who died in one of these facilities.

Who Was Excluded: (1) Records of patients who died as a result of suicide or accident and those who died within 24 hours of admission to the institution or in the emergency department, unless they had been admitted to a VA facility in the preceding month; (2) random selection of patient records were omitted when number of deaths exceeded interviewing capacity; (3) family members who did not speak English or Spanish; (4) family members with a hearing impairment or other health condition that precluded telephone interview; (5) family members who said they could not evaluate the care that the patients received in the last month of life.

How Many Patients: [Family members for] 5,901 decedents.

Study Overview: Surveys contained 10 items: 9 core items measuring specific aspects of care (with frequency-based response options) and the tenth (global) item evaluating the care that the patient received (rating-based response options). Scores were dichotomized, namely for rating-based response options: excellent versus all other responses and for frequency-based response options: best possible response versus all other responses (Figure 5.1).

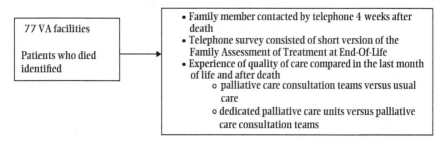

Figure 5.1 Summary of study design.

Study Intervention: Not applicable

Follow-up: Not applicable

Endpoints: Primary outcome was quality of care in dedicated palliative care units compared to palliative care consultation teams in the last month of life and after death. Quality of care was also compared between palliative care consultation teams and usual care.

RESULTS

- 77 VA facilities with both palliative care consultation teams and inpatient palliative care units sampled.
- 5,901 families completed the surveys.
- Response rates were similar in the 2 palliative care groups (66.3% for consultation teams, 64.8% for palliative care unit) but lower in the usual care group (51.3%).
- 2,479 patients died in a palliative care unit, 1,549 received a palliative care consultation, and 1,873 received usual care.
- Comparing palliative care consultations and usual care (Table 5.1):

Table 5.1. SUMMARY OF STUDY'S KEY FINDINGS

Palliative Care Consultations versus Usual Care (Adjusted Mean Scores, %)

	Palliative Care Consultations	Usual Care	OR (95% CI)	P Value
Overall care was excellent	51	46	1.25 (1.02–1.55)	0.04
Providers gave enough spiritual support[a]	52	45	1.36 (1.15–1.61)	0.01
Providers gave enough emotional support before death[a]	57	49	1.35 (1.14–1.60)	0.01

Palliative Care Units versus Palliative Care Consultations (Adjusted Mean Scores, %)

	Palliative Care Consultations	Palliative Care Units	OR (95% CI)	P Value
Overall care was excellent	63	53	1.52 (1.25–1.85)	<0.001
Providers gave enough emotional support before death[a]	67	57	1.53 (1.26–1.86)	<0.001
Providers gave enough spiritual support[a]	62	53	1.45 (1.21–1.73)	<0.001
Providers gave enough emotional support after death[a]	68	59	1.45 (1.18–1.79)	0.001

NOTE: OR = odds ratio; CI = confidence interval.

[a]Specific care items with largest effect size.

- Families of patients who received a palliative care consultation were more likely to report that the overall care that the patient received in the last month of life was excellent.

- Better outcomes were reported by families of patients who received a palliative care consultation for all but 3 items: pain management, assistance with funeral arrangements, and post-death emotional support (no significant differences were found).
- Patients who received a palliative care consultation were more likely to have a do-not-resuscitate order documented at the time of death, a documented chaplain visit, and documented discussion of goals of care in the last month of life. Families of patients who received a palliative care consultation were also more likely to receive a bereavement contact after the patient's death.
- Comparing palliative care units and palliative care consultations:
  - Families of patients who received care in a palliative care unit were more likely to report that the overall care that the patient received in the last month of life was excellent.
  - Better outcomes were reported by families of patients who received care in a palliative care unit for all items except pain management.
  - Patients who received care in a palliative care unit were more likely to have a do-not-resuscitate order documented at the time of death and a documented chaplain visit. They were not more likely to have documented discussion of goals of care in the last month of life, but families of patients who received care in a palliative care unit were more likely to receive a bereavement contact after the patient's death.

Criticisms and Limitations:

- This study is a survey, and not a randomized controlled trial, thus subject to potential bias and confounders.
- Weighting and propensity score adjustments used to account for nonresponse bias and nonrandom assignment rely on accurate measurement of variables of interest, and there is possibility of unmeasured characteristics affecting the results.
- This study was based on survey data of family members of patients who died in specific VA facilities. Thus the decedents were generally older men, which may not be representative of the general US population.
- After patients were identified, family members were contacted 4 weeks after the patient's death. This method resulted in only 52% of identified patients having family members complete the survey. For example, a large number of family members were not eligible for the study for logistical reasons (e.g., unable to be contacted, did not return survey). Others refused or did not have adequate knowledge of the patient's care.

- The survey is largely based on participants' recollection, which may, in the time lapse between the patient's death and survey completion, be less accurate. Recall bias may be a concern. Furthermore, a ceiling effect was observed in family caregivers' perceptions of quality of care.
- The patients who received care from a palliative care consultation team may have received as few as only one consultation, thus limiting the potential benefit.

Other Relevant Studies and Information:

- While many studies report the benefits of palliative care services to patients and family members, the optimal service delivery model is unknown. The literature also focuses largely on palliative care services in the cancer setting.[2–4]
- This is the only study to compare the effect of palliative care consultation teams with that of dedicated palliative care units from a family member's perspective.[1] A study by Gaertner and colleagues further provides evidence to suggest that in particular more complex patients might especially benefit from admission to specialized palliative care units in addition to palliative care consultation.[6]
- Ultimately, the optimal model may be contingent on specific individual (e.g., patient and family preferences, patient's medical condition) and institutional factors (e.g., resource availability). Some authors recommend identifying effective components of palliative care services for integration and implementation based on the resources of individual health care systems and institutions.[4,6,7]

Summary and Implications: In this study, end-of-life care provided by dedicated palliative care units was rated by bereaved family members of deceased patients to be better than that of palliative care consultation teams. Nonetheless, the study also shows that either palliative care model can play a key role in end-of-life care. Effective components of each model need to be identified, and the optimal model needs to be tailored to patients' and family members' needs and preferences, as well as the local resources available.

CLINICAL CASE: WHERE BEST TO PROVIDE END-OF-LIFE CARE?

Case History

A 75-year-old man with metastatic gastric cancer has progressed through several lines of systemic therapies with palliative intent and has no further anticancer treatment options. He is declining rapidly, and his performance status is 4. His symptoms are severe abdominal pain related to his disease site, as well as intermittent nausea and vomiting. He is also fatigued and sleeping most of the day, and his oral intake has diminished considerably. He needs assistance with care including personal hygiene and toileting. He is in the hospital being treated with antibiotics for an intercurrent infection, and this appears to be resolving. His daughter has questions about his ongoing care.

Suggested Answer

This patient with high care needs and high symptom burden would clearly benefit from some form of palliative care service, if not already referred. Moreover, his daughter (and other family members) would also benefit from the assistance with coping and other forms of support: physical, emotional, or spiritual. Referral to palliative care should be discussed with the patient and daughter first and foremost.

Most institutions have developed palliative care consultation teams in order to improve care for patients at the end of life. Internationally there are differences among countries as to the availability of inpatient palliative care units; however, major cancer centers around the world will have access to dedicated inpatient units.

Given this patient is in the hospital, the local resources available for palliative care provision should be discussed, whether this is a palliative care consultation team or a dedicated unit. If there is no inpatient unit option, then the patient and daughter should be reassured of the merits of the palliative care consultation team. However, if there is a dedicated unit, it may be preferable to offer this as an option, noting that some patients will choose to remain in their original setting for reasons such as familiarity with staff and environment.

References

1. Casarett D, Johnson M, Smith D, et al. The optimal delivery of palliative care: a national comparison of the outcomes of consultation teams vs inpatient units. *Arch Intern Med.* 2011 Apr 11;171(7):649–655.

2. Hui D, Bruera E. Models of integration of oncology and palliative care. *Ann Palliat Med.* 2015 Jul;4(3):89–98.

3. Temel JS, Greer JA, Muzikansky A, et al. Early palliative care for patients with metastatic non-small-cell lung cancer. *N Engl J Med.* 2010 Aug 19;363(8):733–742.

4. El-Jawahri A, Greer JA, Temel JS. Does palliative care improve outcomes for patients with incurable illness? A review of the evidence. *J Support Oncol.* 2011 May-Jun;9(3):87–94.

5. Gaertner J, Frechen S, Sladek M, et al. Palliative care consultation service and palliative care unit: why do we need both? *Oncologist.* 2012;17(3):428–435.

6. Luckett T, Phillips J, Agar M, et al. Elements of effective palliative care models: a rapid review. *BMC Health Serv Res.* 2014 Mar 26;14:136.

7. Hui D, Bruera E. Integrating palliative care into the trajectory of cancer care. *Nat Rev Clin Oncol.* 2016 Mar;13(3):159–171.

6

Availability and Integration of Palliative Care at US Cancer Centers

PEDRO PÉREZ-CRUZ AND ALFREDO RODRÍGUEZ-NÚÑEZ

> Despite significant growth in the number of palliative care programs during the past decade, there remains much heterogeneity in the infrastructure and delivery of care in US cancer centers.
>
> —HUI ET AL.[1]

Research Question: What is the availability and degree of integration of palliative care (PC) services in US cancer centers?

Funding: National Cancer Institute (NCI) and the Royal College of Physicians and Surgeons of Canada.

Year Study Began: 2009.

Year Study Was Published: 2010.

Study Location: 1,482 Commission of Cancer (CoC)-accredited cancer centers in the United States.

Who Was Studied: Executives' and PC leaders' perceptions from the CoC-accredited cancer centers.

Who Was Excluded: Not applicable.

How Many Patients: This study was based on number of cancer centers: all 71 NCI-designated cancer centers and a random sample of 71 out of 1,411 non-NCI-designated cancer centers.

Study Overview: The research team generated two surveys to assess the status of PC in cancer centers. One survey was sent to cancer center executives to assess access and attitudes toward PC. A second survey was sent to PC program leaders to describe local program characteristics (Figure 6.1).

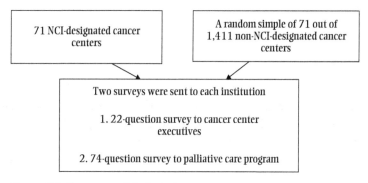

Figure 6.1 Summary of study design.

Study Intervention: Not applicable.

Follow-up: Not applicable.

Endpoints: Primary outcome: Availability of PC services in cancer centers, defined as the presence of at least 1 PC physician.

RESULTS

- The response rate, including complete and partial responses, was 71% (101/142) for executives and 82% (96/117) for PC program leaders. PC program leaders from NCI cancer centers were more likely to respond than program leaders from non-NCI cancer centers (91% [61/67] versus 70% [35/50]; P = .007).

- The availability of PC programs was 98% (50/51) for NCI cancer centers and 78% (39/50) for non-NCI cancer centers ($p = .002$). The PC clinical services available are described in Table 6.1.

Table 6.1. DIFFERENCES IN THE AVAILABILITY OF PC SERVICES BETWEEN NCI AND NON-NCI CANCER CENTERS ACCORDING TO CANCER CENTER EXECUTIVES

PC Services	NCI Cancer Centers (N = 51)			Non-NCI Cancer Centers (N = 50)			
	N	%	95% CI	N	%	95% CI	P Value
Inpatient consultation team	47	92	81–98	28	56	41–70	0.001
Outpatient clinic	30	59	44–72	11	22	12–36	0.001
PC acute care	13	26	14–40	10	20	10–34	0.64
Institution-operated hospice	16	31	19–46	21	42	28–57	0.31

NOTE: PC = palliative care; NCI = National Cancer Institute; CI = confidence interval.

- The most frequent perceived barriers to PC access according to cancer center executives were limited institutional budget, poor reimbursement, and limited training of PC staff.
- Cancer center executives rated their current pain and PC services favorably and reported a significant improvement compared with 5 years prior to the study. NCI cancer center executives were more likely than non-NCI cancer executives to believe that PC personnel funding would increase over the next 5 years (% agree or stronger agree = 44% [22/51] versus 23% [11/50], $p = .03$).
- NCI and non-NCI executives agreed that a stronger integration of PC services into oncology practice will benefit patients and that more funding should be directed toward PC research.
- Most PC teams had physicians (80%), physician assistants (71%), social workers (55%), and nurses (47%). Only one-third of PC program leaders identified their professional background as PC.
- The inpatient consultation teams, outpatient clinics, and PC units were generally larger and served more patients at NCI than at non-NCI cancer centers.
- In general, training and research programs were scarce in both types of institutions. However, NCI cancer centers were more likely to have a PC fellowship than non-NCI cancer centers (38% [23/61] versus 17% [6/65], $p = .04$).

Criticisms and Limitations:

- The number of cancer centers surveyed was limited. The authors only surveyed cancer centers approved by the CoC and did not include any nonaccredited hospitals, which could limit its generalizability.
- PC status among non-NCI cancer centers might be overestimated or underestimated given that only a small percentage was sampled.
- This survey was conducted in 2009. It is unclear what is the current status of cancer centers in the United States.

Other Relevant Studies and Information:

- Over the past years, NCI-designated comprehensive cancer centers in the United States have had an overall trend toward increased supportive care services that focus mainly on pain management services.[2]
- As a parallel to NCI-designated cancer centers, the European Society of Medical Oncology (ESMO) developed a similar approach to define ESMO-designated cancer centers. These institutions have more extensive PC services relative to non-designated cancer centers and urban hospitals, but a minority had inpatient PC beds and institutional supported hospice services. Barriers to PC were similar to those in the United States (i.e., largely financial).[3]
- The goal of integration is to maximize patient access to PC and, ultimately, to improve patient outcomes.[4] To achieve this aim, a group of international experts reached broad consensus on a list of indicators of integration, which may be used to identify centers with a high level of integration and facilitate benchmarking, quality improvement, and research.[5]

Summary and Implications: This study provides a high-level view of the state of palliative care in cancer centers in the United States. It highlights that cancer center executives recognized the importance of pain and PC services at their institutions and that there was an improvement in the availability of these services between 2005 and 2010. This study details that inpatient consultation teams, outpatient clinics, and PC units were generally larger and served more patients at NCI than at non-NCI cancer centers. This study also reveals the relative lack of outpatient clinics, PC units, and community programs, as well as delays in referral for PC services. Finally, this study highlights the need to consolidate infrastructure, to increase the training of PC professionals, to improve research in the field, to educate patients and families, and to advocate for public health challenges in order to attain the American Society of Clinical Oncology's vision of full integration of PC as a routine part of cancer care by 2020.[6]

CLINICAL CASE: WHERE WOULD YOU REFER THIS PATIENT?

Case History

A 56-year-old man with a past medical history of tobacco use visited his primary care physician (PCP) due to a 5 weeks' history of dysphagia, cough, and weight loss. The physical exam was unremarkable. Upper endoscopy showed a mass in the upper third of the esophagus. A thoracic CT suggested the diagnosis of upper esophageal cancer with bilateral thoracic lymph nodes. The PCP explained to the patient that he was probably a candidate for cancer treatment but also that the patient would benefit from PC. What would be the implications for the patient to be referred to a NCI versus a non-NCI cancer center in terms of the availability of PC?

Suggested Answer

In this case the patient would require an integrated approach to cancer treatment, including a medical oncologist, a surgical oncologist, and radiation therapy. Due to the intensity of the interventions, the side effects of the treatments, and the poor prognosis, the patient would definitely benefit from integrating PC early in the trajectory of the disease.

As suggested by the paper by Hui et al., although most cancer centers have PC programs and are strongly supported by their executives, referring the patient to a NCI-designated cancer center increases the patient's likelihood of effectively receiving PC. Also, at a NCI cancer center the patient would be more likely assessed by the PC team, either by the inpatient consultation team or at the outpatient clinic. In both cases, however, the referrals would occur late in the trajectory of the disease, highlighting the pending task of timely integration of PC into standard cancer care.

Due to all these differences, the PCP in this case might check with the cancer centers within the vicinity to understand what palliative care services are available at these institutions increase the likelihood of the patient to receive integrated PC throughout cancer care.

References

1. Hui D, Elsayem A, De La Cruz M, et al. Availability and integration of palliative care at US cancer centers. *JAMA,* 2010;303(11):1054–1061.
2. Hammer SL, Clark K, Grant M, Loscalzo MJ. Seventeen years of progress for supportive care services: a resurvey of National Cancer Institute-designated comprehensive cancer centers. *Palliat Support Care.* 2015;13(4):917–925.

3. Davis MP, Strasser F, Cherny N. How well is palliative care integrated into cancer care? A MASCC, ESMO, and EAPC Project. *Support Care Cancer.* 2015;23(9):2677–2685.

4. Hui D, Bruera E. Integrating palliative care into the trajectory of cancer care. *Nat Rev Clin Oncol.* 2016;13(3):159–171.

5. Hui D, Bansal S, Bruera E, et al. Indicators of integration of oncology and palliative care programs: an international consensus. *Ann Oncol.* 2015;26(9):1953–1959.

6. Ferris FD, Bruera E, Cherny N, et al. Palliative cancer care a decade later: accomplishments, the need, next steps—from the American Society of Clinical Oncology. *J Clin Oncol.* 2009;27(18):3052–3058.

7

Cost Savings Associated with Palliative Care

BREFFNI HANNON

> Our data suggest that palliative care consultation fundamentally shifts
> the course of care off the usual hospital pathway and in doing so, signifi-
> cantly reduces costs.
>
> —MORRISON ET AL.[1]

Research Question: What are the effects of palliative care consultation programs on hospital costs for patients who die in the hospital and for patients who
are discharged from the hospital?

Funding: Center to Advance Palliative Care, the National Palliative Care
Research Center, and a mid-career Investigator award in Patient Oriented
Research.

Year Study Began: 2002.

Year Study Published: 2008.

Study Location: Eight US hospitals, served by 6 palliative care teams. The hospitals were chosen based on their diverse geographical and structural settings and
to represent a variety of socioeconomic demographics.

Who Was Studied: Patients ages 18 years or over who were admitted to the hospital for a period of 7 to 30 days, over a 2-year period from 2002 to 2004.

Who Was Excluded: Initially, patients whose length of stay was fewer than 7 days or more than 30 days. Those with a short length of stay were deemed less likely to receive palliative care; those with a longer length of stay were felt to be outliers who were less representative of the general population. These patients were later included as part of an additional analysis.

Unmatched patients based on propensity scoring were also excluded.

How Many Patients: 43,973 live discharges and 4,726 deaths.

Study Overview: In this retrospective cohort study, each palliative care (PC) patient was matched to at least one usual care (UC) patient based on propensity score. Variables included in the propensity score analysis were age, gender, marital status, medical insurance, primary diagnosis, admitting physician speciality, comorbidity, and intensity of medical services prior to PC involvement. Unmatched patients were excluded (Figure 7.1).

Costs for patients who were seen by the PC consultation team were compared with those who did not see PC (i.e., UC) using hospital administrative data. Databases and billing records were used to identify those patients seen by PC. Patients were stratified based on their disposition (discharged home from hospital versus died in the hospital).

RESULTS

- Patients discharged alive—of the 2,966 patients who received PC and were discharged alive, 2,630 were matched to 18,427 UC patients. PC patients had significantly lower costs than those receiving UC; the net savings (or total cost savings) were \$2,642/admission ($p = 0.02$), or \$279/day ($p < 0.001$). Direct costs (which included costs attributable to intensive care units (ICU), pharmacy, laboratory, and diagnostic imaging) were also significantly lower for the PC group, with savings of \$1,696/admission ($p = 0.004$), or \$174/day ($p < 0.001$). The ICU costs were also significantly lower with PC (\$1,917 vs. \$7,096/admission, $p < 0.001$) (Table 7.1).
- Patients who died in the hospital—2,388 PC patients died in the hospital; 2,278 of these were matched to 2,124 UC patients. Again, there were significant cost savings associated with the PC group, with net total cost savings of \$6,896 per admission ($p = 0.01$), or \$549/day ($p < 0.001$). Direct cost savings were \$4,908/admission ($p = 0.003$), or \$374/day ($p < 0.001$). PC was also associated with lower ICU costs (\$7,929 vs. \$14,542/admission, $p < 0.001$).

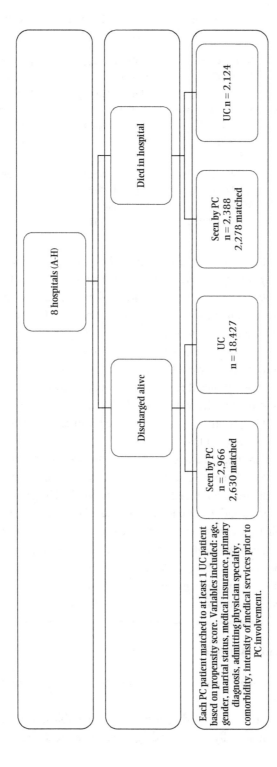

Figure 7.1 Summary of study design.

Table 7.1. Cost Savings Associated with Hospital Palliative Care Consultation Teams

Patient Disposition	Net Savings (Total Costs)	Adjusted Net Savings (Direct Costs)	Direct Costs (including Outliers)
Patients discharged alive	$2,642/admission (P = 0.02) $279/day (P < 0.001)	$1,696/admission (P = 0.004) $174/day (P < 0.001)	<7 days: $275/day >30 days: $246/day
Patients who died in hospital	$6,896/admission (P = 0.001) $549/day (P < 0.001)	$4,908/admission (P = 0.003) $374/day (P < 0.001)	<7 days: $559/day >30 days: 370/day

- Outliers—although initially excluded from the analyses, those patients with a length of stay either <7 days or >30 days were subsequently included. Direct costs were still lower for the PC group; for those discharged alive there was a reduction in cost of $275 (<7 days) and $246 (>30 days). For those who died, the savings were $559 and $370, respectively.
- Confirmatory analyses—the 6 days before and after PC consultation were compared with the overall costs in the UC group. PC was associated with a significant reduction in hospital costs 24 to 48 hours after consultation. For those discharged alive, costs fell from $843 to $605 ($p = 0.001$); for those who died in the hospital, the costs fell from $1,163 to $589, ($p = 0.003$).
- The authors also attempted to estimate what the costs for the PC group would have been if PC had not been consulted. These were not significantly different compared with the costs for the UC group ($p = 0.26$ for live discharges and 0.44 for patients who died in the hospital).
- To ensure that the cost savings seen were not a reflection of a pre-existing change in the treatment plan, mean direct costs for each day of admission for the UC group were plotted against reference days for the PC group. Costs in the PC group were no different until 24 to 48 hours after PC involvement, after which they started to decrease.

Criticisms and Limitations:

- Retrospective analyses were used to generate information about hospital costs.
- Although the authors argued against this, it is possible that referral to the PC team is actually a confounding variable. In the discussions prior

to referring to the PC team, the primary medical team and patient may have agreed upon an altered course of (less aggressive) management, which included referral to PC but would have occurred even in the absence of their involvement. Propensity score analysis may not have taken into account all factors that could influence whether or not patients received PC.

Other Relevant Studies and Information:

- A subsequent prospective, observational study of 5 hospitals (3 of which were included in the current study) demonstrated direct-cost savings associated with early PC referral. Referral within 2 days was associated with the greatest cost savings (24%); referral within 6 days saved up to 14%.[2]
- A meta-review of the economic impact of hospital inpatient PC consultation teams demonstrated the consistent finding of cost savings; less is known about patient and caregiver costs or health systems costs.[3]
- In addition to the timing of referral, cost-saving effects may be influenced by patient complexity. One study has shown savings of up to 22% for patients with comorbidity scores of 3 or lower, rising to 32% for those with comorbidity scores of 4 or higher.[4]

Summary and Implications: In this study, PC was associated with significant cost savings—almost $1,700 for live discharges and $5,000 for patients who died. These results have important implications for hospital administrators. Extrapolating these data to a mid-sized hospital (400 beds) with a PC team seeing 500 patients per year, the estimated annual savings were $1.3 million.

CLINICAL CASE: MAKING A FINANCIAL CASE FOR HOSPITAL-BASED PALLIATIVE CARE TEAMS

Case History

As an administrator for an acute, mid-sized hospital, you are tasked with cutting your clinical budget for the coming year without reducing clinical services or frontline staff. Your hospital serves a community with a growing number of older patients with multiple medical comorbidities and incorporates cancer care services.

Suggested Answer

Older patients with complex medical histories typically have longer inpatient stays, which often include a myriad of investigations and costly treatments. Previous studies of the clinical benefits of palliative care have clearly demonstrated improvements from the patient and caregiver perspective. The Morrison study adds to these findings by demonstrating significant cost savings associated with a palliative care consultation team. These savings were found both for patients who died in the hospital and those who were discharged alive. The authors postulate that this could translate into savings of $1.3 million dollars per year after physician and other personnel costs.

In this case, even the costs of hiring a palliative care consultation team would ultimately be offset by the potential savings. Promoting a culture of early referral of suitable patients to the palliative care team could potentially be associated with even greater savings.

References

1. Morrison RS, Penrod JD, Cassel JB, et al. Cost savings associated with US hospital palliative care consultation programs. *Arch Int Med.* 2008;168(16):1783–1790.
2. May P, Garrido M, Cassel JB, et al. Prospective cohort study of hospital palliative care teams for inpatients with advanced cancer: earlier consultation is associated with larger cost-saving effect. *J Clin Oncol.* 2015;33:2745–2752.
3. May P, Normand C, Morrison RS. Economic impact of hospital inpatient palliative care consultation: review of current evidence and directions for future research. *J Palliat Med.* 2014;17(9):1054–1063.
4. May P, Garrido MM, Cassel JB, et al. Palliative care teams' cost-saving effect is larger for cancer patients with higher numbers of comorbidities. *Health Aff (Millwood)* 2016;35(1):44–53.

Symptom Assessment and Management

8

Changes in the Last Months of Life

JACLYN YOONG AND FIONA RUNACRES

Mean symptom score trajectories followed two patterns: increasing versus generally flat over time. . . . The high proportion of moderate to severe symptom scores in the final weeks of life represents opportunities for improved patient care at the end of life.

—Seow et al.[1]

Research Question: What are the trajectories of symptoms and performance status at the end of life?

Funding: Ontario Institute for Cancer Research and the Institute for Clinical Evaluative Sciences.

Year Study Began: 2007.

Year Study Published: 2011.

Study Location: Ontario, Canada.

Who Was Studied: From January 1, 2007, to March 31, 2009, adult cancer patients registered in the Ontario cancer registry were identified by linkage of multiple administrative health care databases. Patients who died in this study period who had at least one Edmonton Symptom Assessment System (ESAS) or Palliative Performance Scale (PPS) assessment in the last 26 weeks (approximately 6 months) before death were included. Patients were mostly in ambulatory care settings and some home care settings.

Who Was Excluded: Patients who did not die or who did not have an ESAS or PPS recorded in the 26 weeks prior to death.

How Many Patients: 10,752 decedents had at least one ESAS assessment and 7,882 decedents had at least one PPS assessment; 7,508 had both assessments.

Study Overview: Observational cohort study. The study's main objective was to describe the trajectory of ESAS and PPS scores in the last 6 months of life (Figure 8.1).

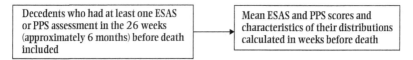

Figure 8.1 Summary of study design.

- ESAS is a patient-reported tool that measures symptom severity, range 0 to 10, where 10 is the worst possible. Severity is categorized as none (0), mild (1–3), moderate (4–6) and severe (7–10); scores ≥4 considered clinically significant. Total Symptom Distress Score (TSDS) is the sum of all symptom scores except for well-being and ranges between 0 and 90.
- PPS is a provider-rated tool measured in 10-point increments, range 0 to 100%, where 100% is best; based on patient's level of ambulation, activity level, evidence of disease, ability to self-care, intake, and level of consciousness.

Study Intervention: Not applicable.

Follow-up: Not applicable.

Endpoints:
- Main outcomes were mean ESAS scores and mean PPS scores per week closer to death.
- Using ESAS, the odds ratio of reporting scores ≥4 (i.e., moderate to severe) for each symptom and the proportion of patients reporting scores ≥4 at each week to death were also analyzed.

RESULTS

- In the last 6 months of life, patients had an average of 5.3 ESAS assessments (standard deviation [SD], 9.7) and an average of 4.9 PPS assessments (SD 8.7) (Table 8.1).

Table 8.1. SUMMARY OF STUDY'S KEY FINDINGS

	26 Weeks Before Death	4 Weeks Before Death	1 Week Before Death
Mean PPS scores	68.4 (SD 14.4)	54.7 (SD 14.2)	41.3 (SD 18.0)
Average TSDS	19.9 (SD 13.4)	28.3 (SD 14.1)	33.6 (SD 14.5)
Mean ESAS: *Unchanged*	Scores did not increase >1 point on ESAS scale over time for pain, nausea, anxiety, depression		
Mean ESAS: *Increased severity*	Scores increased on ESAS scale over time for shortness of breath, drowsiness, well-being, lack of appetite, tiredness		
Symptom scores ≥4 in last month of life	• Less than one-third reported scores ≥4 for all symptoms except nausea • Less than two-thirds reported scores ≥4 for drowsiness, tiredness, well-being, lack of appetite		

Odds of reporting scores ≥4	Symptom	Before the last month of life (OR, 95% CI)	In the last month of life (OR, 95% CI)
	Anxiety	1.02 (1.02–1.03)	1.09 (1.03–1.16)
	Lack of appetite	1.03 (1.02–1.04)	**1.22 (1.14–1.30)**[a]
	Depression	1.03 (1.02–1.03)	**1.09 (1.05–1.19)**[a]
	Drowsiness	1.04 (1.03–1.05)	**1.41 (1.32–1.50)**[a]
	Nausea	1.02 (1.02–1.03)	1.06 (0.98–1.14)
	Pain	1.02 (1.02–1.03)	1.03 (0.97–1.09)
	Shortness of Breath	1.03 (1.02–1.03)	**1.12 (1.06–1.19)**[a]
	Tiredness	1.04 (1.03–1.04)	**1.36 (1.26–1.48)**[a]
	Well-being	1.03 (1.02–1.03)	**1.13 (1.05–1.21)**[a]

NOTE: PPS = Palliative Performance Scale; TSDS = Total Symptom Distress Score; ESAS = Edmonton Symptom Assessment System; SD = standard deviation; OR = odds ratio; CI = confidence interval.

[a] Regression coefficient for change in slope was significant.

- Mean PPS score showed a slight decrease from 26 weeks (mean 68%) to 4 weeks (mean 55%) before death, followed by a more rapid decrease in the last weeks of life (mean 41% in the last week before death).
- For mean symptom scores, two general patterns observed: (1) generally flat over time: nausea, depression, anxiety, pain; overall increased by

no more than 1 point over time; (2) generally increased over the last 6 months of life: shortness of breath, drowsiness, well-being, lack of appetite, tiredness.

- Symptom burden showed a slight increase from 26 (mean TSDS 20) to 4 weeks (mean TSDS 28) before death, followed by a more rapid increase in the last weeks of life (mean TSDS 34 in the last week before death).
- Proportion of patients reporting scores ≥4 at any given week increased closer to death
  - less than one-third reported scores ≥4 for all symptoms except nausea in the last month of life.
  - less than two-thirds reported scores ≥4 for 4 symptoms—drowsiness, tiredness, well-being, lack of appetite—in the last month of life.
- Odds ratio of reporting scores ≥4 per symptom:
  - Increased significantly each week closer to death
    - Before the last month of life: odds increased by 2% to 4% (95% confidence interval [CI], 1.02–1.04)
    - In last month of life: odds increased by (ranging from): 9% (95% CI, 1.05–1.19) for depression to 41% (95% CI, 1.32–1.50) for drowsiness

---

Criticisms and Limitations:

- Patients included in the study were not systematically screened at regular intervals; assessments occurred on an opportunistic basis and not every patient or provider completed the ESAS or PPS tool.
- ESAS in this study assessed symptom intensity "now" (instead of average over 24 hours), which may fluctuate significantly over time.
- The study was limited to an outpatient ambulatory cohort of a cancer center thus is not generalizable to hospitalized patients who are often in greater distress.

Other Relevant Studies and Information:

- The literature is limited in terms of studies that provide this kind of longitudinal symptom and performance status follow-up, and all other studies are small in sample size in comparison. Nonetheless, symptom profiles described in other studies are similar to this study, with nausea largely being the least burden symptom and symptoms such as tiredness, lack of appetite, well-being, and drowsiness showing the least improvement or greatest deterioration over time.[2–5]

Summary and Implications: In this large observational cohort study involving ambulatory patients, symptom trajectories in the last 6 months of life followed two general patterns: increasing or generally flat. A high proportion of patients also reported moderate to high severity of symptoms in the last month of life, and performance status declined rapidly toward the end of life. These findings offer insights about how to counsel patients toward the end of life and how end-of-life care might be improved.

CLINICAL CASE: WHAT TRAJECTORY OF SYMPTOMS CAN BE ANTICIPATED TOWARD THE END OF LIFE?

Case History

A 75-year-old man with metastatic non-small cell lung cancer has tumor-related chest pain and shortness of breath from a mild-moderate pleural effusion and newly diagnosed pulmonary emboli. He is concerned about his current symptoms and how they will progress as he becomes more unwell. He is also wondering about other symptoms that may develop over time. What should he be told?

Suggested Answer

The patient wants to know what to expect as his disease progresses. People want to know this for different reasons (e.g., wanting to know how their symptoms may affect their functioning and what they can continue doing; some fear debilitating symptoms that may lead to intractable suffering and worry about their sense of independence; others want to better understand their illness, how to prepare and what practical things can be done to manage anticipated symptoms). These reasons are important to explore in order to counsel the patient appropriately and provide information that is relevant and constructive to the patient, especially given that some symptoms are likely to worsen over time.

Based on the results of this study, the patient can be counseled that these are symptoms commonly experienced by cancer patients. He should be advised that while each case is individual (depending on site of disease, complications, and perception of symptoms), the literature does suggest some patterns of symptomatology. For example, pain appears largely stable over time, potentially due to availability of effective interventions. However, shortness of breath may be less well controlled; and strategies to deal with this, for now and in the future, may be discussed. The patient can also be informed of other possible symptoms such as tiredness, drowsiness, and lack of appetite that may be less amenable to intervention; however, he should also be told that these symptoms, together with declining performance status, only appear to be most prominent in the last month of life.

The oncologist should discuss a referral to palliative care services (if not already done) to help improve quality of life and to proactively manage his symptoms, either with medications, psychosocial support, or possibly practical supports.

References

1. Seow H, Barbera L, Sutradhar R, et al. Trajectory of performance status and symptom scores for patients with cancer during the last six months of life. *J Clin Oncol.* 2011 Mar 20;29(9):1151–1158.
2. Barbera L, Seow H, Howell D et al. Symptom burden and performance status in a population-based cohort of ambulatory cancer patients. *Cancer.* 2010 Dec 15;116(24):5767–5776.
3. Yennurajalingam S, Urbauer DL, Casper KL et al. Impact of a palliative care consultation team on cancer-related symptoms in advanced cancer patients referred to an outpatient supportive care clinic. *J Pain Symptom Manage.* 2011 Jan;41(1):49–56.
4. Zeng L, Zhang L, Culleton S et al. Edmonton Symptom Assessment Scale as a prognosticative indicator in patients with advanced cancer. *J Palliat Med.* 2011 Mar;14(3):337–342.
5. Strasser F, Sweeney C, Willey J et al. Impact of a half-day multidisciplinary symptom control and palliative care outpatient clinic in a comprehensive cancer center on recommendations, symptom intensity, and patient satisfaction: a retrospective descriptive study. *J Pain Symptom Manage.* 2004 Jun;27(6):481–491.
6. Walsh D, Donnelly S, Rybicki L. The symptoms of advanced cancer: relationship to age, gender, and performance status in 1,000 patients. *Support Care Cancer.* 2000 May;8(3):175–179.

9

The Edmonton Symptom Assessment System

BREFFNI HANNON

> The ESAS is a simple and useful method for the assessment of palliative care patients.
>
> —BRUERA ET AL.[1]

Research Question: Patient self-assessment tools are considered the gold standard for the assessment and management of cancer distress. Many such assessment tools are laborious and time-consuming for patients to complete or expensive for practitioners to access outside of clinical trials settings, however. This study aimed to report the use of a single-page, visual analog scale (VAS), the Edmonton Symptom Assessment System (ESAS), as part of routine clinical care on a palliative care unit.

Funding: Unspecified.

Year Study Began: Unspecified.

Year Study Published: 1991.

Study Location: Palliative Care Unit at Edmonton General Hospital, Alberta, Canada.

Who Was Studied: Consecutive patients with advanced cancer admitted to the palliative care unit.

Who Was Excluded: Unspecified.

How Many Patients: 101.

Study Overview: This was an open, prospective study assessing the feasibility of using a symptom assessment tool as part of routine clinical care on an inpatient palliative care unit. All inpatients completed the ESAS independently if able; alternatively, they could be assisted by a nurse, the nurse could independently complete the ESAS, or a family member could complete it if the patient was unable or unwilling.

Study Intervention: The ESAS is a single-page VAS with eight 100mm domains assessing the following physical and psychological symptoms: pain, activity, nausea, depression, anxiety, drowsiness, appetite, and well-being. An additional space is available for any symptom(s) outside of this list that the patient wishes to report. The scores are logged and transferred to a graph, which allows for the rapid visual review of symptoms for up to 21 days on a single page. The ESAS was administered twice daily (at 10.00 and 18.00) to all patients admitted consecutively to the palliative care unit. Scores were graphed and summed to form an overall ESAS Distress Score with a maximum of 800mm.

Follow-up: Twice daily follow-up.

Endpoints: Unspecified.

RESULTS

- 6,352 assessments were completed for 101 patients over 3,352 patient days
- Distress score results were compared for Days 1 to 5 following admission; results were significantly lower at Day 5 compared with Day 1 (Table 9.1).
- 84% of patients completed the ESAS independently upon admission; ultimately 96% required nurse completion and 4% family member completion as the patients' clinical status deteriorated.
- Mean distress scores when the ESAS was completed by the patient alone, patient assisted by a nurse, nurse alone, and family member were compared (Table 9.2).

Table 9.1. DISTRESS SCORES DAYS 1–5 FOLLOWING ADMISSION

Day from Admission	N	Distress Score (Mean and SD)	P Value
Day 1	101	410 +/–95	—
Day 3	97	367 +/–97	Nonsignificant
Day 5	95	362 +/–83	<0.01

NOTE: SD = standard deviation.

Table 9.2. COMPARISON OF DISTRESS SCORES BASED ON PERSON COMPLETING THE ESAS

ESAS Completed By	ESAS Distress Score (Mean and SD)	P Value
Patient	359+/–105	—
Patient assisted by nurse	374 +/–93	Nonsignificant
Nurse	359 +/–91	Nonsignificant
Family member	406 +/–81	<0.01

NOTE: ESAS = Edmonton Symptom Assessment System; SD = standard deviation.

- Family members were more likely to report higher distress scores than patients or nurses (P < 0.01).

Criticisms and Limitations:

- This was a single-center study of a newly developed VAS symptom assessment system.
- As one of the first symptom assessment batteries, ESAS was not psychometrically derived and was not validated against an existing symptom assessment tool in the original study. Information about user feedback was limited.
- Exclusion criteria were not specified and the length of follow-up was unclear.
- No information was given about the time anchor (assumed to be "now") and the optional ninth symptom, including how often additional symptoms were added and what these symptoms were.

Other Relevant Studies and Information:

- Other commonly used symptom assessment tools include the Memorial Symptom Assessment System (MSAS).[2]

- Further studies have validated the ESAS against the MSAS and other questionnaires.[3,4] Compared with the MSAS, the ESAS is shorter and considered easier to complete from a patient perspective.
- The ESAS is now typically presented as a numerical rating scale rather than a VAS and assesses the average symptom intensity of the past 24 hours.[4,5]
- A variation of the ESAS (called the ESAS-r) asks about symptom intensity "now" and includes additional symptoms such as shortness of breath, tiredness, and drowsiness; while activity has been removed.[6]
- The ESAS has been validated in a number of different languages as well as for use in nonmalignant patient populations.[5]
- A recent prospective study identified the minimal clinically important difference for ESAS was 1 point for both improvement and deterioration for all items.[7]
- The ESAS has been adopted as the standardized symptom screening tool for all cancer patients across Ontario, Canada, since 2006, in conjunction with symptom management guidelines and algorithms. Over 28,000 unique patient reports are collected monthly, with screening rates reported as quality indicators for each regional cancer centre.[8]

Summary and Implications: This prospective study demonstrated that the ESAS is a useful, acceptable tool for routine symptom assessment among seriously ill patients admitted to a palliative care unit. The publication of this manuscript paved the way for further validation of this scale in both cancer and noncancer populations. The ESAS is now available in over 20 languages and is used for both patient care and research worldwide.[9]

CLINICAL CASE: THE UTILITY OF SYMPTOM ASSESSMENT SYSTEMS FOR COMPLEX PATIENTS AND FAMILIES

Case History

A 60-year-old man is referred to the palliative care team shortly after his diagnosis of stage IV non-small cell lung cancer. His wife and daughter have been phoning the team regularly reporting a constellation of physical and psychological symptoms, but the patient himself is reluctant to make any changes to his medications.

Suggested Answer

Since symptoms are a truly subjective phenomenon, patient-reported symptom assessment tools are the gold standard. The Bruera study showed that family members are more likely to report higher symptom burden compared to patients' own reports as well as nurse-assisted or independent nurse reports. Relying on family reports of symptom burden may lead to overtreatment of symptoms and increase the risks of adverse drug effects.

The routine use of the ESAS allows for health care providers to track symptoms over time and to objectively assess the response to prescribed treatments. It may also have a role in helping patients to become more involved in their health care, acting as a prompt for discussion points with their health care teams.

References

1. Bruera E, Kuehn N, Miller MJ, Selmser P, MacMillan K. The Edmonton Symptom Assessment System: a simple method for the assessment of palliative care patients. *J Palliat Care*. 1991;7(2):6–9.
2. Porteney RK, Thaler HT, Kornblith AB, et al. The Memorial Symptom Assessment Scale: an instrument for the evaluation of symptom prevalence, characteristics and distress. *Eur J Cancer*. 1996;30A:1226–1236.
3. Chang T, Huang SS, Feuerman M. Validation of the Edmonton Symptom Assessment Scale. *Cancer*. 2000;88:2164–2171.
4. Hannon B, Dyck M, Pope A, et al. Modified Edmonton Symptom Assessment System including constipation and sleep: validation in patients with cancer. *J Pain Symptom Manage*. 2015;49(5):945–952.
5. Nekolaichuk C, Watanabe S, Beaumont C. The Edmonton Symptom Assessment System: a 15-year review of validation studies (1991–2006). *Palliat Med*. 2008;22:111–122.
6. Watanabe S, Nekolaichuk C, Beaumont C, Johnston L, Myers J, Strasser F. A multicenter validation study of two numerical versions of the Edmonton Symptom Assessment System in palliative care patients. 2011. *J Pain Symptom Manage*. 2011;41:456–468.
7. Hui D, Shamieh O, Paiva CE, et al. Minimal clinically important differences in the Edmonton Symptom Assessment Scale in cancer patients: a prospective, multicenter study. *Cancer*. 2015;121(17):3027–3035.
8. Pereira J, Green E, Molloy S, et al. Population-based standardized symptom screening: Cancer Care Ontario's Edmonton Symptom Assessment System and performance status initiatives. *J Oncol Pract*. 2014 May;10(3):212–214.
9. Hui D, Bruera E. The Edmonton Symptom Assessment System 25 years later: past, present, and future developments. *J Pain Symptom Manage*. 2017;53(3):630–643.

10

Reversibility of Delirium in Palliative Care

TIFFANY SHAW AND ERIC PROMMER

> Despite its terminal presentation in most patients, delirium is reversible in approximately 50% of episodes.
>
> —LAWLOR ET AL.[1]

Research Question: What are the precipitating causes, degree of reversibility, and impact of delirium on prognosis?

Funding: Cantel-Overton Fellowship, University of Alberta, Edmonton (Dr. Gagnon) and the Institut Jules Bordet, Unite Bruxelles, Brussels, Belgium (Dr. Mancini).

Year Study Began: Patient accrual occurred from February 1 through October 19, 1997. In-hospital follow-up ended in January 1998.

Year Study Published: 2000.

Study Location: Tertiary level, acute palliative care unit (APCU) at Grey Nun's Hospital, a university-affiliated teaching hospital in Edmonton, Alberta.

Who Was Studied: Patients with advanced cancer and delirium.

Who Was Studied: Consecutive patients with a histologic diagnosis of cancer admitted to a APCU. Patients with dementia were included.

Who Was Excluded: Patients with psychiatric disorders interfering with delirium assessment. Inability to speak English or communicate because of cancer-related complications led to exclusion.

How Many Patients: 113 acute consecutive patient admissions with 104 patients meeting eligibility criteria. Nine patients were excluded for reasons such as language, tracheostomies, expressive dysphasia, depressive psychosis, and family wishes. Thirty-three patients without delirium were used as a control group.

Study Overview: Investigators screened for cognitive deficit by obtaining a Mini-Mental State Examination (MMSE) on all patients on admission, twice weekly, and at any time if the onset of delirium was suspected. Attending palliative care physicians also assessed patients twice daily during the weekdays and once daily at weekends.

Once delirium was diagnosed according to *Diagnostic and Statistical Manual of Mental Disorders* (fourth edition) criteria, regular assessment of delirium severity and symptoms was conducted using the Memorial Delirium Assessment Scale (MDAS) and a semistructured interview (twice in the first 72 hours of delirium and once every 72 hours thereafter for as long as delirium persisted). Investigators documented total daily opioid dose, expressed as subcutaneous morphine equivalent daily dose. Patients with clinical evidence of opioid toxicity underwent opioid dose reduction or change of opioid. Patients with clinical or laboratory evidence of dehydration received hydration using hypodermoclysis. Patients with infection received appropriate oral or intravenous antibiotics according to patient and family wishes. Patients with hypercalcemia received subcutaneous clondronate or intravenous pamidronate disodium. All patients with a diagnosis of delirium received regular neuroleptic therapy and midazolam if unresponsive to neuroleptics (Figure 10.1).

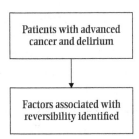

Figure 10.1 Summary of study design.

Intervention: Not applicable.

Follow-up: 1 to 47 days.

Endpoints: Delirium occurrence, reversibility of delirium patient survival.

RESULTS

- On admission, delirium was diagnosed in 44 patients (42%) (Table 10.1).
- In 60 patients, delirium developed in 27 (45%) over the course of admission.

Table 10.1. SUMMARY OF UNIVARIATE ANALYSES OF PRECIPITATING FACTOR
CATEGORIES ASSOCIATED WITH REVERSIBILITY OF DELIRIUM

Categories	Reversed (%)	Irreversible (%)	Hazard Ratio (95% CI)	P Value
Psychoactive drugs	38 (95)	15 (48)	8.85 (2.13–36.7)	0.003
Dehydration	26 (95)	8 (26)	2.35 (1.20–4.62)	0.01
Hematologic	5 (13)	7 (23)	0.58 (0.22–1.51)	0.25
Nonrespiratory infection	10 (25)	8 (26)	0.56 (0.26–1.18)	0.12
Metabolic	10 (25)	18 (58)	0.44 (0.21–0.91)	0.02
Hypoxic encephalopathy	11 (28)	22 (71)	0.39 (0.19–0.80)	0.008
Miscellaneous other causes	7 (18)	7 (23)	0.69 (0.30–1.59)	0.37

NOTE: CI = confidence interval.

- Reversal of delirium occurred in 46 (49%) of 94 episodes in 71 patients.
- Terminal delirium occurred in 46 (88%) of the 52 deaths.
- The median number of precipitating factors was 3 (range = 1–6).
- In univariate analysis, psychoactive medications, chiefly opioids (HR, 8.85) and dehydration (HR, 2.35), were associated with reversibility. Hypoxic encephalopathy (HR, 0.39) and metabolic factors (HR, 0.44) were associated with nonreversibility.
- In multivariate analysis, psychoactive medications (HR, 6.65), hypoxic encephalopathy (HR, 0.32), and nonrespiratory infection (HR, 0.23; 95% confidence interval, 0.08–0.64) had independent association with reversibility of delirium.
- Patients with delirium had poorer survival rates than controls ($P < 0.001$).

Criticisms and Limitations:

- Because this is a study of cancer patients admitted to an acute palliative care unit, the study findings may not be generalizable to other populations. Specifically, patients in this study had high symptom burden, high nurse–patient and physician–patient ratios, and low rates of dementia.
- The frequency of delirium severity assessments was limited in this study in an effort not to impose undue burden on terminally ill patients. Fluctuations in the MDAS scoring could be explained by fluctuations in delirium per se as opposed to the effects of treatment of various causes.
- The study was unable to examine the role of environmental stresses that could have contributed to the development of delirium.

Other Relevant Studies and Information:

- Leonard and coworkers[2] evaluated factors related to reversibility of delirium in palliative care patients experiencing delirium. Investigators used the Delirium Rating Scale and Cognitive Test for Delirium for delirium rating. Patients with irreversible delirium had shorter survivals and higher delirium instrument scores. Irreversible delirium was associated with greater disturbances in speech, sleep, long-term memory and attention, vigilance, and visuospatial function. Older patients and those with organ failure were likely to die sooner than those with reversible delirium.

Summary and Implications: The study represents the first analysis of precipitating factors in developing delirium. The study highlights the need to diagnose delirium and to recognize both its multifactorial nature and reversibility. Systematic use of screening tools such as the MMSE and rating tools such as the MDAS may facilitate the diagnosis of delirium. The identification of reversible factors allows the physician to use low-burden therapies such as opioid switching and/or dose modification, discontinuation or dose reduction of other psychotropic medications, and hydration with hypodermoclysis (common term for the subcutaneous infusion of fluids in hospice setting) to reverse delirium, even in patients with a short survival.

CLINICAL CASE: DOES THIS PATIENT HAVE A REVERSABLE CAUSE OF DELIRIUM?

Case History

A 73-year-old man with advanced head and neck cancer (HPV negative) is being evaluated for control of delirium. The patient required emergent airway control due to obstructing tumor and experienced a prolonged hypoxic episode. Upon reawakening the patient experienced hyperactive delirium refractory to nonpharmacologic and pharmacologic (neuroleptics) interventions. A member of the palliative care team asks whether or not his delirium will improve.

Suggested Answer

The presence of hypoxic encephalopathy increases the risk for irreversible delirium. Looking for reversible causes in a systematic way is indicated. The presence of refractory delirium may require other pharmacologic interventions designed to improve the comfort of the patient. Communication with family or other health care proxies should convey the likelihood of a short prognosis.

References

1. Lawlor PG, Gagnon B, Mancini IL, et al. Occurrence, causes, and outcome of delirium in patients with advanced cancer: a prospective study. *Arch Intern Med.* 2000;160:786–794.
2. Leonard M, Raju B, Conroy M, et al. Reversibility of delirium in terminally ill patients and predictors of mortality. *Palliat Med.* 2008;22:848–854.

11

Multicomponent Intervention to Prevent Delirium in Hospitalized Older Patients

PETER LAWLOR

> This controlled clinical trial provides evidence that a multicomponent, targeted intervention strategy, the Elder Life Program, is effective for the prevention of delirium in hospitalized older medical patients.
>
> —INOUYE ET AL.[1]

Research Question: What is the comparative effectiveness of a targeted multicomponent strategy for reducing the risk of delirium with that of usual standard care for hospitalized older patients? Also, what is the level of adherence to the strategy's protocol and how effective is it in reducing the targeted risk factors for delirium?

Funding: National Institute on Aging, the Commonwealth Fund, the Retirement Research Foundation, the Community Foundation for Greater New Haven, and the Patrick and Catherine Weldon Donaghue Medical Research Foundation.

Year Study Began: 1995.

Year Study Published: 1999.

Study Location: Yale New Haven Hospital, a teaching hospital, New Haven, CT.

Who Was Studied: Patients 70 years old or greater who were consecutively admitted to the general medical service (nonintensive care) without delirium at the time of admission.

Who Was Excluded: Those with profound dementia, language barrier, aphasia, intubation or respiratory isolation, coma or terminal illness, hospital stay ≤ 48 hours, prior enrollment, and patient or family refusal to consent.

How Many Patients: 852.

Study Overview: This was a prospective matched cohort study. Computerized matching with a 1:1 ratio was used for eligible patients admitted to the intervention unit versus those admitted to two usual care units. Matching was based on age, sex, and baseline risk of delirium. The baseline risk of delirium was determined by the presence of risk factors previously identified in an empiric study. The risk was classified as intermediate (1 to 2 risk factors) or high (3 to 4 risk factors) (Figure 11.1).

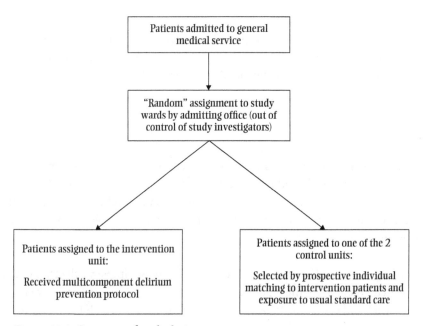

Figure 11.1 Summary of study design.

Study Intervention: Eligible patients in the intervention unit received a nonpharmacologic multicomponent intervention strategy that aimed to prevent delirium by targeting six risk factors: cognitive impairment, sleep deprivation, immobility, visual impairment, hearing impairment, and dehydration. At baseline, there was standardized assessment of risk factors by researchers who had no role in applying targeted interventions and were blinded as to the group assignment and the nature of the study. The targeted interventions were delivered by a trained interdisciplinary team of specialist nurses, a geriatrician, a physiotherapist, a recreational therapist, and trained volunteers.

Follow-up: Until hospital discharge at a median of 7.0 and 6.5 days in the intervention and control groups, respectively.

Endpoints: Primary outcome: delirium in both groups, based on daily cognitive testing and Confusion Assessment Method (CAM) ratings, recorded as incidence, total person-days in delirium, number of episodes, severity of episodes, and recurrence rate of delirium in both groups. Secondary outcomes: status of risk factors at Day 5 of admission in both groups and level of adherence to intervention protocol.

RESULTS

- In the intervention group, 42/426 (9.9%) had a first incident episode of delirium compared to 64/426 (15%) in the usual care group (Table 11.1).

Table 11.1. SUMMARY OF STUDY'S KEY FINDINGS

Outcomes Analyses	Intervention Group (n = 426)	Usual Care Group (n = 42)	P Value
All patients (N = 852)			
First incident episode of delirium: n (%)	42 (9.9)	64 (15)	0.02[a]
Total patient-days of delirium	105	161	0.02[b]
No. of episodes of delirium	62	90	0.03[b]
Patients with delirium (n = 106)			
Delirium severity score: mean ± SD	3.85 ± 1.27	3.52 ± 1.44	0.25[c]
Patients with recurrent (≥ 2 episodes) of delirium: n (%)	13 (31.0)	17 (26.6)	0.62[d]

NOTE: SD = standard deviation.

[a]Odds ratios: 0.6 (95% confidence interval [CI], 0.39–0.92) in matched (conditional logistic regression) and 0.61 (95% CI, 0.40–0.93) in unmatched (standard logistic regression adjusted for matching factors) analyses; P = 0.02 for both. [b]Applying sign test to within pair differences in matched analyses. [c]Using the t-test in an unmatched comparison. [d]Using the chi-square test in unmatched comparison.

- The total number of days with delirium (105 vs. 161) and the total number of episodes (62 vs. 90) were significantly lower in the intervention group.
- The severity of delirium and its recurrence rates were not significantly different in the two study groups, suggesting that the interventional benefit is limited to primary prevention.
- The overall adherence rate for the interventions was 87%. The total number of targeted risk factors per patient was significantly reduced.
- There was significant improvement from baseline in cognitive impairment and significant reduction in the use of sedative drugs for sleep in the intervention group.

Criticisms and Limitations:

- The low delirium rates may reflect contamination across study groups, which would bias toward the null hypothesis, thus perhaps rendering the findings even more significant.
- The overall study mortality of 1.5%, its exclusion of terminally ill patients, and its inclusion of only 6% of the study sample with a cancer diagnosis limit generalizability to other populations, such as younger patients or those at risk of terminal irreversible delirium in the last days/weeks of life.
- This is not a randomized trial—and thus difference in other unmatched variables (e.g., other risk factors for delirium) between groups may contribute to differences; however, the groups were comparable on all 20 measured variables at baseline, indicating the strength of the study design and matching variables.
- Although there was an overall reduction in the incidence of first delirium in the intervention group, a subgroup analysis, based on delirium risk (intermediate or high) revealed a statistically significant reduction in the intermediate baseline delirium risk group but not in the high baseline risk group, where power was limited. This may limit the generalizability of the study findings, especially to high-risk patients in palliative care settings.[2]

Other Relevant Studies and Information:

- Other multicomponent interventional strategies to prevent delirium in hospitalized elderly patients[3-5] have also proven successful, though underlying frailty may attenuate these benefits.[2]

- Multicomponent interventions similar to those in the current study are used in the Hospital Elder Life Program for Prevention of Delirium (HELP). These HELP interventions have been reported to be effective across various patient populations (e.g., surgical, emergency department) and settings (e.g., community hospitals, postacute and long-term care), as well as in other countries (e.g., Australia, Netherlands, Taiwan).[6] Although HELP has also been implemented in some palliative care units, published data are lacking. Subsequent analysis of this study found that a higher level of adherence to the study interventions was associated with greater reduction of delirium.[7]
- A cohort study in palliative care failed to show a reduction in delirium in association with a multicomponent delirium prevention strategy, though this study suffered from methodological limitations.[8]
- Although antipsychotics have been the mainstay of pharmacological management of delirium in palliative care settings, emerging data concerning both their efficacy and safety make a compelling case to better evaluate preventative strategies in such patients.[9]

Summary and Implications: This prospective matched cohort study evaluating a nonpharmacologic multicomponent delirium prevention strategy demonstrated a 30% reduction in the incidence of a first delirium episode within an elderly medical population. Subgroup analysis showed the reduction to be most pronounced among patients with intermediate, rather than high, baseline delirium risk, which may limit the generalizability of this study's findings to high-risk patients, including many in palliative care settings.

At the same time, it is important to note that some palliative care patients (especially those with longer survival) will fall into the intermediate risk group and have reversible risk factors that can be addressed through these nonpharmacologic approaches. Recent data have raised concerns regarding both the efficacy and the safety of antipsychotics in the management of delirium, which makes a compelling case for further rigorously designed studies to better evaluate the role of nonpharmacologic preventative strategies in reducing delirium in palliative care settings.

CLINICAL CASE: WHAT IS THE RISK OF DELIRIUM AND HOW CAN WE PREVENT IT IN A PALLIATIVE CARE UNIT?

Case History

A 72-year-old man with no history of cognitive impairment was recently diagnosed with metastatic non-small cell lung cancer and started on low-dose morphine for painful rib metastases. He refused chemotherapy and radiation therapy. He now presents to the emergency department with a 3-day history of increasing dyspnoea, daytime drowsiness, insomnia, and disorientation to place only; attention span is normal and his overall cognitive impairment does not yield a CAM positive rating for delirium. He is admitted to an inpatient acute palliative care unit for intravenous antibiotic treatment of a pneumonia. What is the risk of delirium in this patient and how can we prevent it?

Suggested Answer

This patient is clearly at risk of delirium, based on his age, cancer diagnosis, and now an intercurrent pneumonia. His mild symptoms of disorientation and drowsiness might indicate a subsyndromal delirium or even prodromal delirium (if we assume that he might go on to actually develop delirium). His drowsiness may be associated with a fluid deficit. His wife is concerned about his insomnia and requests that he receive night time sedation.

Based on the seminal study by Inouye et al. and subsequent literature data,[1,4–6] we should primarily target this patient's prodromal symptoms, albeit mild and not currently reaching the threshold of delirium diagnosis. Regular reorientation efforts, a room with a visible clock, and a board with the names of care-team members are all likely to be helpful in preventing a full delirium. Second, early and regular mobilization as tolerated should be encouraged. In this regard, urinary catheterization is an impediment to mobility and should be avoided if possible. Third, assisted hydration with intravenous or subcutaneous fluids will also have a preventative role. Fourth, his insomnia is initially best treated in a nonpharmacological manner, following a sleep enhancement protocol with optimal sound, lighting, minimized nocturnal interruptions, massage, relaxation music, and a warm drink (e.g., warm milk or herbal tea).

Collectively, these four preventative interventions may help to prevent an episode of incident delirium in this patient who has at least an intermediate risk of delirium. This will help to optimize this patient's quality of life, which is the fundamental goal of palliative care.

References

1. Inouye SK, Bogardus ST Jr, Charpentier PA, et al. A multicomponent intervention to prevent delirium in hospitalized older patients. *N Engl J Med*. 1999;340(9):669–676.
2. Teale E, Young J. Multicomponent delirium prevention: not as effective as NICE suggest? *Age Ageing*. 2015;44(6):915–917.
3. Martinez F, Tobar C, Hill N. Preventing delirium: should non-pharmacological, multicomponent interventions be used? A systematic review and meta-analysis of the literature. *Age Ageing*. 2015;44(2):196–204.
4. Hshieh TT, Yue J, Oh E, et al. Effectiveness of multicomponent nonpharmacological delirium interventions: a meta-analysis. *JAMA Intern Med*. 2015;175(4):512–520.
5. Siddiqi N, Harrison JK, Clegg A, et al. Interventions for preventing delirium in hospitalised non-ICU patients. *Cochrane Database Syst Rev*. 2016;3:Cd005563.
6. Boockvar KS, Teresi JA, Inouye SK. Preliminary data: an adapted hospital elder life program to prevent delirium and reduce complications of acute illness in long-term care delivered by certified nursing assistants. *J Am Geriatr Soc*. 2016 May;64(5):1108–1113
7. Inouye SK, Bogardus ST Jr, Williams CS, Leo-Summers L, Agostini JV. The role of adherence on the effectiveness of nonpharmacologic interventions: evidence from the delirium prevention trial. *Arch Intern Med*. 2003 Apr 28;163(8):958–964.
8. Gagnon P, Allard P, Gagnon B, Merette C, Tardif F. Delirium prevention in terminal cancer: assessment of a multicomponent intervention. *Psychooncology*. 2012;21(2):187–194.
9. Agar MR, Lawlor PG, Quinn S, et al. Efficacy of oral risperidone, haloperidol, or placebo for symptoms of delirium among patients in palliative care: a randomized clinical trial. *JAMA Intern Med*. 2017 Jan 1;177(1):34–42.

12

Haloperidol, Chlorpromazine, and Lorazepam for Delirium

ANNA CECILIA TENORIO AND MAXINE DE LA CRUZ

> Symptoms of delirium [among patients with AIDS] may be treated efficaciously with few side effects by using low dose neuroleptics.
> —BREITBART ET AL.[1]

Research Question: Are neuroleptics more effective and safer than benzodiazepines in treating delirium in hospitalized patients with AIDS?

Funding: National Institute of Mental Health Grant MH-45664.

Year Study Began: Not specified.

Year Study Published: 1996.

Study Location: St. Luke's Roosevelt Hospital Center.

Who Was Studied: Medically hospitalized adults who met the case definition of AIDS undergoing treatment for AIDS-related medical problems at the St. Luke's Roosevelt Hospital Center and who were medically stable with the capacity to give informed consent.

Who Was Excluded: Excluded were patients who had underlying cognitive impairment or diagnosed delirium, those who lacked the capacity to give informed consent, patients with known adverse effects to neuroleptics or benzodiazepines, those already on neuroleptics and benzodiazepines for the treatment of other medical or psychiatric conditions or undergoing current systemic chemotherapy for Kaposis' sarcoma, and patients who had delirium that was determined to be part of a terminal event.

How Many Patients: 30.

Study Overview: This is a double-blind randomized controlled trial in which hospitalized AIDS patients who developed delirium were randomized to receive haloperidol, chlorpromazine, or lorazepam in a 1:1:1 ratio. Patients consented for the study and were monitored every hour using the Delirium Rating Scale (DRS), the Mini Mental State Examination (MMSE), and the Extrapyramidal Symptom Rating scale until delirium was confirmed. Delirious patients then received one of the three study medications. The lorazepam arm was discontinued after only 6 patients because of significant treatment-limiting side effects (Figure 12.1).

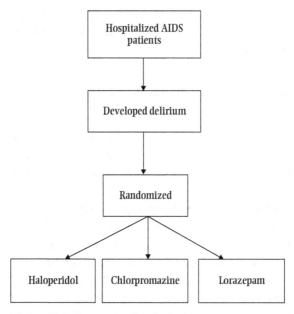

Figure 12.1 Summary of study design.

Study Intervention: Titration phase: once enrolled in the study, patients were assessed hourly with the DRS and the dose of medication continued to increase hourly until patients were asleep, calm, and had hallucinations or had a DRS score of 12 or below.

- Haloperidol starting at 0.25 mg PO (or 0.125 mg IM), titrated over 9 dose levels to a maximum of 5 mg PO (or 3 mg IM)
- Chlorpromazine starting at 10 mg PO (or 5 mg IM), titrated over 9 dose levels to a maximum of 200 mg PO (or 100 mg IM)
- Lorazepam starting at 0.5 mg PO (or 0.2 mg IM), titrated over 9 dose levels to a maximum of 4 mg PO (or 2 mg IM)

Maintenance dose started on Day 2 for up to 6 days. The dose was equal to one-quarter of the first 24-hour total dose given twice.

Follow-up: 6 days.

Endpoints: Primary outcome: Improvement in delirium symptoms as measured using the DRS.

Secondary outcomes: Improvement in cognitive status as measured using the MMSE; development of side effects (extrapyramidal side effects using Extrapyramidal Symptom Rating Scale and monitoring/observation of treatment limiting side effects).

RESULTS

- Improvement in delirium symptoms and cognition in the haloperidol and chloromazine arms was more significant between baseline to Day 2, but there was little or no improvement from Day 2 until the end of treatment (Tables 12.1 and 12.2).
- Lorazepam had no effect on the delirium symptoms and cognition at any point in the study, and it worsened symptoms in the treatment of delirium in AIDS patients when used as a primary agent.
- All 6 patients in the lorazepam group developed treatment-limiting side effects that included oversedation, disinhibition, ataxia, and worsening confusion resulting in drug discontinuation.
- None of the patients receiving the neuroleptics developed dystonic or dyskinetic symptoms during the treatment period.

Table 12.1. SUMMARY OF STUDY'S KEY FINDINGS

	Baseline Mean (SD)	Day 2 Mean (SD)	End of Treatment Mean (SD)	P Value Baseline to Day 2	P Value Day 2 to End of Treatment
Delirium Rating Scale[a]					
Haloperidol	20.45 (3.45)	12.45 (5.87)	11.64 (6.10)	<0.001	<0.43
Chlorpromazine	20.62 (3.88)	12.08 (6.50)	11.85 (6.74)	<0.001	<0.81
Lorazepam	18.33 (2.58)	17.33 (4.18)	17.00 (4.98)	<0.63	<0.81
Cognitive Status (Mini Mental State)[b]					
Haloperidol	13.45 (6.95)	17.27 (8.87)	17.18 (12.12)	<0.09	<0.96
Chlorpromazine	10.92 (10.43)	18.31 (10.61)	15.08 (10.43)	<0.001	<0.04
Lorazepam	15.17 (5.31)	12.67 (10.23)	11.50 (8.69)	<0.40	<0.60

NOTE: SD = standard deviation.

[a] Delirium Rating Scale is a 10-item scale. A score of 13 and above signifies delirium. Maximum score of 32. [b] Mini-Mental State assesses orientation and cognitive capacity. A score of 23 and below is the cutoff for cognitive impairment. Maximum score of 30.

Table 12.2. MEAN AND MAINTENANCE DRUG DOSES

	Mean Dose in the First 24 Hours in mg (SD, Range)	Average Maintenance Doses Day 2 To End of Treatment in mg (SD, Range)
Haloperidol	2.8 (2.4, 0.8–6.3)	1.4 (1.2, 0.4–3.6)
Chlorpromazine	50.0 (23.1, 10–70)	36.0 (18.4, 10.0–80.0)
Lorazepam	3.0 (3.6, 0.5–10.0)	4.6 (4.7, 1.3–7.9)

NOTE: SD = standard deviation.

Criticisms and Limitations:

- The sample size was small, and no sample size calculation was reported.
- The lorazepam arm was terminated early, and it was thus difficult to conclusively evaluate the risks and benefits of lorazepam alone for delirium. Furthermore, no placebo control was included.
- The generalizability of this study was limited by its single-center design and enrollment of only patients with AIDS.
- The survival of this patient population was not reported, making it difficult to know how sick the patients were.
- It was unclear whether the dosing titration approach was optimal since it has not been compared to the scheduled approach directly.

Other Relevant Studies and Information:

- A Cochrane Systematic Review in 2012[2] examining the evidence of drug therapy for delirium in terminally ill patients concluded that this was the only trial that met the inclusion criteria, highlighting the paucity of research in this setting.
- A recent randomized controlled trial that enrolled patients with mild to moderate delirium reported that haloperidol and risperidone were worse than placebo in controlling delirium symptoms and suggested that they be reserved for treating patients with severe agitated delirium.[3]
- Another randomized controlled trial compared a single dose of lorazepam and haloperidol vs. placebo and haloperidol as rescue for severe refractory agitation. Lorazepam and haloperidol was found to significantly reduce agitation and to improve patient's comfort as perceived by caregivers and nurses.[4]

Summary and Implications: This is the first randomized controlled trial to examine pharmacologic interventions for managing delirium in a terminally ill population. It found that neuroleptics were superior to lorazepam. Based on this study, many clinicians concluded that benzodiazepines should not be used in delirium due to excessive harm. Twenty years later, a larger randomized trial has raised questions about these findings, highlighting the need for further studies.

CLINICAL CASE: WHEN SHOULD WE START MANAGING DELIRIUM IN PATIENTS?

Case History

A 58-year-old man with metastatic lung cancer presents to the emergency room with confusion, hallucinations, agitation, and uncontrolled pain. He has a fluctuating level of consciousness. The daughter is particularly concerned about his worsening restlessness and yelling episodes over the past week. He is admitted and found to be obtunded at times and agitated at others. How should we manage this delirium?

Suggested Answer

This patient presents with mixed delirium. It is important to identify and treat any underlying conditions that could have led to the delirium symptoms, such as hypercalcemia, opioid-induced neurotoxicity (due to chronic opioid use), and metabolic abnormalities. Nonpharmacologic measures such as orientation cues and environmental control are also important.

Given that this patient has significant agitation, pharmacologic therapy may be warranted. According to the Breitbart study, patients may potentially benefit from neuroleptics, such as haloperidol (Haldol) or chlorpromazine. Although these medications may induce significant side effects, their use may be justified in this setting for a patient with severe delirium symptoms despite standard measures.

References

1. Breitbart B, Marotta R, Platt M, et al. A double-blind trial of haloperidol, chlorpromazine and lorazepam in the treatment of delirium in hospitalized AIDS patients. *Am J of Psychiatry*. 1996 Feb;153(2):231–237.
2. Candy B, Jackson KC, Jones L, Leurent B, Tookman A, King M. Drug therapy for delirium in terminally ill adult patients (Review). *Cochrane Database Syst Rev*. 2012;11:CD004770. doi:10.1002/14651858.CD004770.pub2
3. Agar MR, Lawlor PG, Quinn S, et al. Efficacy of oral risperidone, haloperidol, or placebo for symptoms of delirium among patients in palliative care: a randomized clinical trial. *JAMA Intern Med*. 2017 Jan 1;177(1):34–42.
4. Hui D, Frisbee-Hume S, Wilson A, Dibaj SS, Nguyen T, De La Cruz M, Walker P, Zhukovsky DS, Delgado-Guay M, Vidal M, Epner D, Reddy A, Tanco K, Williams J, Hall S, Liu D, Hess K, Amin S, Breitbart W, Bruera E. Effect of Lorazepam With Haloperidol vs Haloperidol Alone on Agitated Delirium in Patients With Advanced Cancer Receiving Palliative Care: A Randomized Clinical Trial. *JAMA*. 2017 Sep 19;318(11):1047–1056.

13

Decompressive Surgery for Malignant Spinal Cord Compression

ESMÉ FINLAY AND DIAA OSMAN

> The best treatment for spinal cord compression caused by metastatic cancer is surgery as initial treatment followed by radiotherapy.
> —PATCHELL ET AL.[1]

Research Question: Is direct decompressive surgery plus postoperative radiotherapy superior to radiotherapy alone for treatment of metastatic epidural spinal cord compression (MESCC)?

Funding: National Cancer Institute (R01 CA55256) and National Institute for Neurological Disorders and Stroke (K24 NS502180).

Year Study Began: 1992.

Year Study Published: 2005.

Study Location: Multi-institutional, Bluegrass Neuro-Oncology Consortium (academic medical centers in the United States).

Who Was Studied: Adults with biopsy-proven malignancy, not of central nervous system or spinal column origin, with magnetic resonance imaging (MRI) evidence of MESCC and the following characteristics:

- At least one neurological sign or symptom
- Paraplegia if duration prior to study entry <48 hours
- MESCC restricted to one region
- Expected survival >/= 3 months and fit enough for surgery

Who Was Excluded: Patients with multiple areas of MESCC; patients with certain radiosensitive tumour types; patients with pre-existing or concomitant neurological issues (e.g., brain metastases); patients with prior spinal radiation in affected region.

How Many Patients: 101 randomized; study stopped early because predetermined criteria for early termination were met.

Study Overview: This randomized, multi-institutional, unblinded study compared outcomes between patients with MESCC who received decompressive surgery followed by radiation to those who received radiation alone. Patients were stratified based on institution, tumor type, ability to walk at presentation, and spinal stability. All patients received full-spine MRI evaluation and were treated with high-dose dexamethasone at the time of diagnosis until the study intervention was initiated (Figure 13.1).

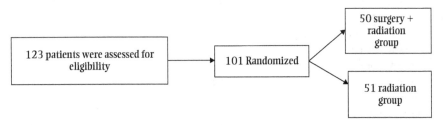

Figure 13.1 Summary of study design.

Study Intervention: Patients randomized to radiation alone started treatment within 24 hours of randomization. Radiation was administered in 10 fractions × 3Gy for a total dose of 30Gy. Patients in the surgery arm received surgical decompression within 24 hours of randomization; the surgical technique was not prespecified. Radiation was provided using the same regimen as in the radiation-only arm and started within 14 days of surgery.

Follow-up: Every 4 weeks until death or the end of the trial.

Endpoints: Primary endpoint: Ability to walk after treatment, with ambulatory rate defined as percentage of participants who "maintained or regained" the ability to walk and ambulatory time defined as the length of time ambulation was maintained posttreatment. Secondary endpoints: Urinary continence, Frankel functional scale score, American Spinal Injury Association motor score, corticosteroid use, opioid use, and survival time.

RESULTS

- Patients randomized to decompressive surgery and radiation had better rates and prolonged duration of ambulation compared to those who had radiation alone, improved rates of urinary continence, improved functional ability, higher muscle strength, longer survival, and a reduction in corticosteroid use (1.6mg of dexamethasone vs. 4.2mg) and opioid analgesics after treatment (0.4mg vs. 4.8mg) (Table 13.1).

Table 13.1. SUMMARY OF STUDY'S KEY FINDINGS

	Radiation Group	Surgery Group	Relative Risk	P Value
Days of maintained ambulatory ability	13d	122d	NA	0.03
Days of maintained continence	17d	156d	0.47	0.016
Days of maintained muscle strength (ASIA score)	72d	566d	0.28	0.001
Days of maintained functional ability (Frankel score)	72d	566d	0.24	0.0006
Survival time	100d	126d	0.60	0.033
Total daily corticosteroid use	4.2mg	1.6mg	NA	NA
Mean morphine equivalent dose	4.8mg	0.4mg	NA	NA

NOTE: d = days; ASIA = American Spinal Injury Association.

- Based on the data, the authors concluded that in appropriately selected patients with a single area of MESCC who were surgical candidates, the combination of spinal decompressive surgery and radiation was better than radiation alone.

Criticisms and Limitations:

- The criteria by which patients were deemed fit enough to be surgical candidates, and therefore candidates for entry into this trial, were not well defined.
- Limited information is provided regarding comorbidities of the enrolled patients.
- Patients with multiple sites of metastasis, those who were paraplegic >48 hours, and patients with known brain metastasis were excluded, as were those with radiosensitive tumours such as from lymphomas, multiple myelomas, or seminomas. Therefore, the study results are not generalizable to these populations.
- This study was conducted in several academic medical centers. Despite the fact that MESCC is an oncologic emergency, patients in the community, especially in rural or underserved regions, may not have immediate access to neurosurgical specialists and radiation services within 24 to 48 hours of diagnosis.

Other Relevant Studies and Information:

- Using matched-pair analysis, another retrospective cohort study among patients with metastatic cancer to the spine comparing surgery + radiation versus radiation alone also demonstrated better outcomes in the surgical group.[2]
- Two meta-analyses reviewed studies completed prior to 2013 comparing patients who received surgery +/− radiation versus those who received radiation alone for spinal metastatic disease. Despite limitations, these results suggest that decompressive surgery and radiation combined result in improved ambulation and survival for patients with MESCC compared to radiation alone.[3,4]
- A prospective study of patients with a single MESCC lesion assessed the impact of surgery on health-related quality of life (HRQoL), clinical, and survival outcomes. Results indicate that patients who had surgery had improvement in many pain, functional, and HRQoL outcomes.[5]

Summary and Implications: This practice-changing study demonstrated that in appropriately selected patients with MESCC, combined decompressive surgery plus radiation improved outcomes, including survival, maintenance of continence, and functional ability, compared to radiation alone. This study has not been replicated on a larger scale, but for appropriately selected patients with

MESCC who have adequate functional reserve, greater than 3-month prognosis, and limited burden of systemic disease, surgery followed by radiation should be considered.

CLINICAL CASE: WHO SHOULD BE REFERRED TO PALLIATIVE CARE?

Case History

A 63-yeawr-old woman with metastatic breast cancer presents to her oncologist for routine oncologic followup complaining of increased pain in the mid-thoracic spine. She describes pain that has progressively worsened over the last 3 weeks, is exacerbated by coughing and walking, and improves slightly with opioids. Her Eastern Cooperative Oncology Group Perfomance Status is 2. On physical exam she has point tenderness over the T8/T9 vertebral bodies.

Urgent MRI reveals an expansive bony metastasis in the T8 vertebral body displacing the spinal cord, associated with spinal cord edema. She has another small T2 lesion that is not associated with any cord compression. Recent restaging scans reveal a low burden of systemic disease. Should she be referred to a neurosurgeon and/or a radiation oncologist for management of this spine lesion?

Suggested Answer

Yes, she should be referred urgently to a neurosurgeon and radiation oncology to reduce her risk of progressive morbidity from this spine lesion. She ideally should be managed with dexamethasone followed by immediate surgery if her performance status and comorbidities do not exclude her as a surgical candidate. Surgery should be followed by external-beam radiation therapy. A multidisciplinary approach is best to ensure coordinated, appropriately timed treatments, with goals of maintaining function, reducing pain, and prolonging her life.

References

1. Patchell RA, Tibbs PA, Regine WF, et al. Direct decompressive surgical resection in the treatment of spinal cord compression caused by metastatic cancer: a randomised trial. *Lancet.* 2005;366(9486):643–648. doi:10.1016/S0140-6736(05)66954-1
2. Rades D, Huttenlocher S, Dunst J, et al. Matched pair analysis comparing surgery followed by radiotherapy and radiotherapy alone for metastatic spinal cord compression. *J Clin Oncol.* 2010;28(22):3597–3604. doi:10.1200/JCO.2010.28.5635

3. Lee C-H, Kwon J-W, Lee J, et al. Direct decompressive surgery followed by radiotherapy versus radiotherapy alone for metastatic epidural spinal cord compression: a meta-analysis. *Spine*. 2014;39(9):E587–E592. doi:10.1097/BRS.0000000000000258

4. Klimo P, Thompson CJ, Kestle JRW, Schmidt MH. A meta-analysis of surgery versus conventional radiotherapy for the treatment of metastatic spinal epidural disease. *Neuro-Oncol*. 2005;7(1):64–76. doi:10.1215/S1152851704000262.

5. Fehlings MG, Nater A, Tetreault L, et al. Survival and clinical outcomes in surgically treated patients with metastatic epidural spinal cord compression: results of the prospective multicenter AOSpine study. *J Clin*. 2016;34(3):268–276. doi:10.1200/JCO.2015.61.9338

14

Opioid Rotation for Toxicity Reduction

ANNA CECILIA TENORIO AND AKHILA REDDY

> Opioid toxicity can be relieved by opioid rotation, and a choice of 2-3 different opioids is necessary to obtain satisfactory long-term pain control.
>
> —DE STOUTZ ET AL.[1]

Research Question: Opioid toxicity may develop due to accumulation of metabolites following chronic opioid use. Does opioid rotation reduce dose-limiting toxicities among patients who are on chronic opioid treatment for cancer pain? Also, what is the impact of opioid rotation on pain control?

Funding: None.

Year Study Began: 1991.

Year Study Published: 1995.

Study Location: Edmonton General Hospital Palliative Care Unit (EGH-PCU).

Who Was Studied: Consecutive sample of patients who were admitted at the Edmonton General Hospital Palliative Care Unit between April 1, 1991, and October 1, 1992.

Who Was Excluded: Patients who did not undergo opioid rotation.

How Many Patients: 80.

Study Overview: This was a retrospective review of a consecutive sample of patients with advanced cancer admitted to EGH-PCU. Patients who acquired dose-limiting toxicities with opioids and subsequently underwent opioid rotation (substitution of one opioid with another) were studied (Figure 14.1). Dose-limiting toxicity symptoms were defined as cognitive failure, hallucinations, uncontrolled pain, myoclonus, nausea, and local irritation. Pain was scaled based on the Edmonton Staging for Cancer Pain scale, which is a pain staging according to mechanism of pain, pain characteristics, previous use of opioids, cognitive function, psychological distress, tolerance to pain medication, and history of addiction.[2] Pain was measured as part of the Edmonton Symptom Assessment System, which is a (0–10) visual analog scale of pain and 8 other symptoms.[3]

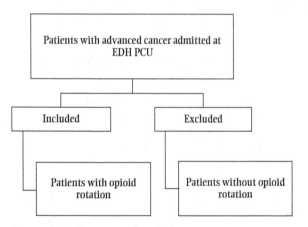

Figure 14.1 Summary of study design.

Study Intervention: Opioid rotation.

Follow-up: The 24-hour new opioid doses were calculated after 3 days of titration for all opioids and 5 to 7 days for methadone.

Endpoints: Improvement of symptoms, namely cognitive failure, hallucinations, pain, myoclonus, and nausea. These outcomes were assessed by chart review of notes and other quantitative records.

RESULTS

- 80 patients out of 191 underwent opioid rotation. Total number of opioid rotations were 111; however, only the first opioid rotation in patients who underwent more than one rotation was included in the analysis.
- Morphine was the most frequently used opioid prior to opioid rotation. Indeed, 53 of the 80 opioid rotations were from morphine to hydromorphone.
- As compared to the patients who did not undergo opioid rotation, at baseline the patients who underwent opioid rotation had more difficult pain syndromes, longer palliative care unit stay (37 days vs. 22 days; P = 0.0001), and higher dose of opioid (morphine equivalent daily dose [MEDD] 578 vs. 250 mg).
- Cognitive failure (43%) was the most common indication for opioid rotation followed by hallucinations (24%), uncontrolled pain (16%), myoclonus (11%), nausea (9%), and local irritation (1%).
- MEDD decreased significantly after opioid rotation (P = 0.04) (Table 14.1).
- Opioid rotation resulted in improvement of pain, cognitive failure, hallucinations, myoclonus, and nausea (Table 14.2).

Table 14.1. OUTCOME: BEFORE AND AFTER OPIOID ROTATION – ALL PATIENTS (N = 80)

	Before Opioid Rotation	After Opioid Rotation	P Value
MEDD (mg)	577 (+/−1535)	336 (+/−593)	0.04
MMS	18 (+/−10)	21 (+/−9)	0.04
Pain VAS	4.4 (+/−2.3)	3.6 (+/−2)	0.004

NOTE: MEDD = morphine equivalent daily dose; MMS = Mini Mental State Questionnaire; VAS = visual analog scale.

Table 14.2. SYMPTOM IMPROVEMENT AFTER OPIOD ROTATION ACCORDING TO THE LEADING SYMPTOM[a]

	Improvement
Leading symptom improvement	58/80 (73%) P = <0.01
Cognitive failure	29/42 (66%) P < 0.01
Hallucinations	10/15 (67%) P = NS
Myoclonus	9/9 (100%) P < 0.002
Pain	7/10 (70%) P = NS
Nausea	2/4 (50%) P = NS

NOTE: NS = nonsignificant.

[a]Leading symptom is the main reason for opiod rotation identified in the patient's chart.

Criticisms and Limitations:

- Patients were found to have clinical significant improvement in leading symptoms after opioid rotation; however, co-interventions addressing factors that may also contribute to symptom burden (e.g., fluids for dehydration, antibiotics for infections, reversal of electrolyte abnormalities, deprescribing of psychotropic medications) were not reviewed.
- The study was also a retrospective study, which depended mostly on medical and nursing documentation to evaluate symptom improvement.
- Renal failure was found in 16 patients (20%) patients but not subjected to subgroup analysis.
- The sample size was relatively small and did not allow for separate analysis of different combinations of opioids involved in the process of opioid rotation.

Other Relevant Studies and Information:

- Studies have shown that opioid rotation is beneficial in both inpatient and outpatient settings and can be performed safely to manage uncontrolled pain or opioid induced neurotoxicity in cancer patients not responding to titration of opioids.[4,5]
- Previous studies have shown that the most common indication for opioid rotation in the outpatient setting is uncontrolled pain, and in the inpatient setting it is opioid induced neurotoxicity.[4,5]
- Several studies have shown that methadone is the most common opioid that is being used for opioid rotation with a 77% success rate in the inpatient setting and an 84% success rate in the outpatient setting.[5]
- Although opioid rotation is now an established tool for managing uncontrolled cancer-related pain or opioid-induced neurotoxicity, the practice is not in widespread use due to a lack of established safe opioid rotation ratios and clinician inexperience.[6,7]

Summary and Implications: This is the first study to establish that opioid rotation can be safely and effectively used to treat uncontrolled pain and opioid-induced neurotoxicity. Multiple studies have subsequently been published supporting opioid rotation for symptom management.

CLINICAL CASE: WHAT TYPE OF PATIENTS SHOULD UNDERGO OPIOID ROTATION?

Case History

The patient is a 63-year-old man with metastatic renal cell carcinoma to the spine who presented to the clinic with uncontrolled pain and signs of mild jerking. The patient and his wife deny any hallucinations, confusion, nausea, or memory impairment. The patient takes a total of morphine extended release 100 mg tablets 3 times daily (MEDD: 300). Morphine was discontinued immediately and the patient was advised to start long-acting hydromorphone 32mg tablet daily, with short-acting hydromorphone 4mg every 4 hours as needed for breakthrough pain. Follow-up in 48 hours revealed significant pain improvement and disappearance of jerking (myoclonus).

Suggested Answer

The patient presented with uncontrolled symptoms concerning for opioid-induced neurotoxicity. Based on the Stoutz study, patients with these types of symptoms would benefit from opioid rotation, by substituting equianalgesic doses of a different opioid medication. The patient in this case improved significantly with the rotation to hydromorphone. This case exemplifies the safety and efficacy of opioid rotation in the outpatient setting.

References

1. de Stoutz N, Bruera E, Suarez-Almazor M. opioid rotation for toxicity reduction in terminal cancer patients. *J Pain Symptom Manage.* 1995 July 5;10(5):378–384.
2. Bruera E, MacMillan K, Hanson J, MacDonald RN. The Edmonton Staging System for Cancer Pain: preliminary report. *Pain.* May 1989;37(2):203–209.
3. Bruera E, Kuehn N, Miller MJ, Selmser P, Macmillan K. The Edmonton Symptom Assessment System (ESAS): a simple method for the assessment of palliative care patients. *J Palliat Care.* 1991;7(2):6–9.
4. Mercadante S, Ferrera P, Villari P, Casuccio A, Intravaia G, Mangione S. Frequency, indications, outcomes and predictive factors of opioid switching in an acute palliative care unit. *J Pain Symptom Manage.* 2009 Apr 4;37(4):632–641.
5. Reddy A, Yennurajalingam S, Pulivarthi K, et al. Frequency, outcome and predictors of success within 6 weeks of an opioid rotation among outpatient with cancer receiving strong opioids. *Oncologist.* 2013;18:212–220.

6. Webster LR, Fine PG. Review and critique of opioid rotation practices and associated risks of toxicity. *Pain Med.* 2012;13(4):562–570.

7. Bruera E, Pereira J, Watanabe S, Belzile M, Kuehn N, Hanson J. Opioid rotation in
patients with cancer pain: a retrospective comparison of dose ratios between methadone, hydromorphone, and morphine. *Cancer.* 1996;78(4):852–857.

15

Duloxetine for Chemotherapy-Induced Peripheral Neuropathy

REBECCA BURKE AND AKHILA REDDY

> Among patients with painful chemotherapy-induced peripheral neuropathy, the use of duloxetine . . . resulted in a greater reduction in pain.
> —SMITH ET AL.[1]

Research Question: Is duloxetine more effective than placebo in decreasing chemotherapy-induced peripheral neuropathic pain (CIPN)?

Funding: National Cancer Institute (NCI) Division of Cancer Prevention, the Alliance Statistics and Data Center, and the Alliance Chairman. Drug and placebo were supplied by Eli Lilly.

Year Study Began: 2008.

Year Study Published: 2013.

Study Location: 8 NCI-funded cooperative research networks.

Who Was Studied: Patients 25 years and older receiving paclitaxel, another taxane, or oxaliplatin at a community or academic setting with grade 1 or higher sensory neuropathy according to National Cancer Institute (NCI) Common Terminology Criteria for Adverse Events (CTCAE) and average chemotherapy-induced pain score of at least 4/10.

Who Was Excluded: Patients with a documented medical history of neuropathy from any type of nerve compression, leptomeningeal carcinomatosis, severe depression, suicidal ideation, bipolar disease, alcohol abuse, a major eating disorder, or markedly abnormal renal or liver function tests were excluded.

How Many Patients: 231.

Study Overview: This is a randomized, double-blind, placebo-controlled crossover trial in which 231 eligible patients were randomized using a 1:1 ratio, then stratified by chemotherapeutic drug and comorbid risk (Figure 15.1).

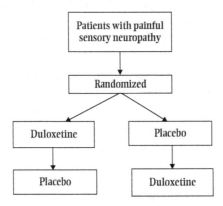

Figure 15.1 Summary of study design.

Study Intervention: Patients were allocated to group A or B. Group A received duloxetine 60mg daily as initial treatment and placebo as crossover treatment. Group B received placebo as initial treatment and duloxetine as crossover treatment. Initial weeks (1–5) and crossover weeks (8–12) each consisted of either 30mg duloxetine or one capsule placebo for the first week, then 60mg duloxetine or 2 capsules placebo for 4 weeks, then a 2-week washout period commenced. Total study duration was 14 weeks.

Follow-up: 5 weeks.

Endpoints: Primary outcome: change in average pain severity using the Brief Pain Inventory–Short Form. Secondary outcomes: change in chemotherapy-induced peripheral neuropathy–related quality of life using the Functional Assessment of Cancer Therapy (FACT)/Gynecologic Oncology Group Neurotoxicity subscale (GOG-NTX), change in degree of pain interference with daily function using the Brief Pain Inventory–Interference score and adverse events using the NCI CTCAE version 3.0.

RESULTS

- At the end of the initial treatment period, patients in the duloxetine-first group reported a statistically significant decrease in the mean pain score compared to the placebo-first group (1.06 vs. 0.34; P = 0.003; Table 15.1).
- The mean difference in average pain score between duloxetine-first and placebo-first groups was 0.73.
- Patients who had received platinums for chemotherapy experienced more benefit from duloxetine than those that received taxanes.
- Compared to placebo, patients treated with duloxetine first reported a greater decrease in the amount of pain that interfered with daily functioning (P = 0.01).
- Pain-related quality of life improved to a greater degree for those treated with duloxetine first.
- No hematologic, moderately severe, or severe adverse events were reported.
- Fatigue, insomnia, and nausea were the most common adverse events reported by patients treated with duloxetine.

Table 15.1. SUMMARY OF STUDY'S KEY FINDINGS

	Duloxetine-First Group	Placebo-First Group
Change in pain score[a]	1.06	0.34
Change in pain interference with daily function score[a]	7.9	3.5
Change in chemotherapy induced peripheral neuropathy related quality of life[b]	2.44	0.87
% decrease in numbness/tingling in feet	41	23

[a] Per Brief Pain Inventory score. [b] Per Functional Assessment of Cancer Therapy (FACT)/Gynecologic Oncology Group Neurotoxicity subscale (GOG-NTX) score.

Criticisms and Limitations:

- More patients receiving duloxetine dropped out of the study due to adverse effects as compared to placebo (11% vs. 1%; P < 0.001).
- While this study included a geographically diverse group of patients, it excluded patients with abnormal liver function tests and kidney disease, limiting the generalizability of the findings.

Other Relevant Studies and Information:

- This article reviewed 15 NCI-supported clinical trials testing effective treatments for chemotherapy-induced peripheral neuropathy. Duloxetine was the only drug proven to have therapeutic benefit.[2]
- This study confirmed the safety and efficacy of duloxetine for treatment of diabetic peripheral neuropathy compared to placebo.[3]
- A literature review found evidence to support venlafaxine and duloxetine for the treatment of CIPN from oxaliplatin- or paclitaxel-based drugs but noted that no direct comparison studies were available between the two drugs.[4]

Summary and Implications: CIPN is a difficult condition to treat. This well-designed study is the first large phase 3 trial to demonstrate the effectiveness of an intervention for treating painful CIPN. Duloxetine is now considered the gold standard for this condition.

CLINICAL CASE: WHO SHOULD BE STARTED ON DULOXETINE?

Case History

A 67-year-old male with a past medical history of carcinoma of the bladder is status posttreatment with cisplatin and radical cystectomy. He achieved remission of his cancer but has suffered from daily burning and tingling pain in his lower extremities since completion of chemotherapy. He rates the pain as 8/10 on numerical rating scale. He is no longer able to enjoy daily walks in the park with his wife secondary to the constant pain in his legs.

Would you consider starting duloxetine to treat CIPN in this patient?

Suggested Answer

The Smith trial demonstrated that patients experiencing painful CIPN experienced a statistically significant decrease in pain score and improvement in function and quality of life with duloxetine therapy compared to placebo.

This patient is experiencing cisplatin-induced painful neuropathy that interferes with his ability to function in daily activities. The pain is interfering with his quality of life and causing significant pain burden. A conversation should be held with the patient discussing the possible benefits of initiating duloxetine therapy, as well as a discussion of the risks associated with the addition of any medication. Fortunately, duloxetine specifically has been shown to be relatively well tolerated with minimal side effects.

References

1. Smith EM, Pang H, Cirrincione C, et al. Effect of duloxetine on pain, function, and quality of life among patients with chemotherapy-induced painful peripheral neuropathy: a randomized clinical trial. *JAMA*. 2013 Apr 3;309(13):1359–1367. doi: 10.1001/jama.2013.2813. PubMed PMID: 23549581; PubMed Central PMCID: PMC3912515

2. Majithia N, Temkin SM, Ruddy KJ, Beutler AS, Hershman DL, Loprinzi CL. National Cancer Institute-supported chemotherapy-induced peripheral neuropathy trials: outcomes and lessons. *Support Care Cancer*. 2016 Mar;24(3):1439–1447. doi: 10.1007/s00520-015-3063-4. Review. PubMed PMID: 26686859; PubMed Central PMCID: PMC5078987

3. Raskin J, Pritchett YL, Wang F, D'Souza DN, Waninger AL, Iyengar S, Wernicke JF. A double-blind, randomized multicenter trial comparing duloxetine with placebo in the management of diabetic peripheral neuropathic pain. *Pain Med*. 2005 Sep-Oct;6(5):346–356. PubMed PMID: 16266355

4. Aziz MT, Good BL, Lowe DK. Serotonin-norepinephrine reuptake inhibitors for the management of chemotherapy-induced peripheral neuropathy. *Ann Pharmacother*. 2014 May;48(5):626–632. doi: 10.1177/1060028014525033. Review. PubMed PMID: 24577146

16

Effects of Morphine on Dyspnea

ARIF H. KAMAL AND JASON A. WEBB

SC morphine controls dyspnea at doses that do not compromise respiratory function.

—BRUERA ET AL.[1]

Research Question: How does tailored doses of morphine affect dyspnea scores and respiratory parameters in patients with advanced cancer?

Funding: Not reported.

Year Study Began: 1988.

Year Study Published: 1990.

Study Location: Single center, palliative care unit.

Who Was Studied: Adults age >18 years of age, with advanced cancer and severe dyspnea at rest due to restrictive respiratory failure and supplemental oxygen dependent

Who Was Excluded: Children, non-cancer patients, primary reason for dyspnea related to obstruction (obesity, chronic obstructive pulmonary disease).

How Many Patients: 20.

Study Overview: This study was an open-label, single arm pilot study of tailored subcutaneous (SC) morphine doses on dyspnea and pain scores (Figure 16.1).

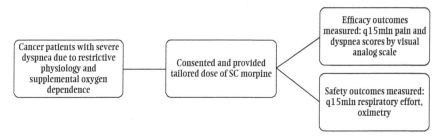

Figure 16.1 Summary of study design.

Study Intervention: Tailored SC morphine dose.

Follow-up: Measurements of efficacy and safety occurred every 15 minutes for a total 150 minutes. All 20 patients completed all assessments.

Endpoints: Primary outcomes were visual analog scale (VAS) dyspnea and pain scores. Secondary outcomes involve respiratory effort (measured by respiratory rate) and oximetry.

RESULTS

- Dyspnea scores, measured at 15-minute intervals, improved significantly at 45 minutes after SC morphine administration compared to baseline.
- No significant adverse side effects were reported related to respiratory effort and oxygenation parameters (Table 16.1).

Table 16.1. SUMMARY OF STUDY'S KEY FINDINGS

	Before Morphine	45 Minutes After Morphine	P Value
Dyspnea (VAS measured 0–10 at q15m intervals)	68 ± 32	34 ± 25	<0.001
Saturation of O2	87 ± 10	86 ± 11	NS

NOTE: VAS = visual analog scale; O2 = oxygen; NS = nonsignificant.

Criticisms and Limitations:

- Since there was no control group, it is not possible to know how morphine therapy compared with other forms of therapy or no therapy at all.
- The study was a small pilot study only involving patients with cancer, indicating a need for future controlled studies in broader populations to make more definitive conclusions.

Other Relevant Studies and Information:

- Subsequent placebo-controlled, double-blind randomized trials and systematic reviews support the efficacy of opioids for palliation of dyspnea in cancer and non-cancer patients.[2–5]

Summary and Implications: This is one of the first prospective studies to suggest that opioids can be used to relieve dyspnea in patients with advanced cancer without also causing hypoxemia as a side effect. Subsequent research stimulated by this study has confirmed the benefits of opioids for managing distressing symptoms at the end of life.

CLINICAL CASE: SHOULD THIS ADVANCED CANCER PATIENT WITH DYSPNEA BE TREATED WITH MORPHINE?

Case History

A 57-year-old woman with stage IV (pleural lining, spleen, omentum) ovarian cancer is admitted to the palliative care service for severe dyspnea related to an expanding pleural effusion. Significant pleural caking by metastatic disease has made continued pleural drainage very difficult; the most recent thoracentesis only produced 100mL of straw-colored fluid. She reports dyspnea at rest, a VAS score of 8/10, and minimal exertion for the past 6 weeks. Supplemental nasal cannula oxygen as high as 6L continuously has not helped much. She is receiving maximal medical management, including bronchodilators and small doses of diuretics. She does not require opioids for management of cancer pain.

What other medication may ameliorate the dyspnea of this patient?

Suggested Answer

The small pilot study by Bruera et al. highlights the important role of opioids in the management of dyspnea refractory to supplemental oxygen therapy in patients with advanced cancer. In addition to finding a significant and dramatic decrease by cumulative dyspnea score over 45 minutes by half, the authors observed no decrements in usual respiratory parameters after one dose of SC morphine. In addition to the obvious pain benefits of morphine, the results of this pilot study suggest an important role of doses of morphine tailored to the previous experiences of an individual patient with opioids (naïve vs. tolerant) in ameliorating dyspnea. A trial of 5mg of SC morphine may be warranted as adjuvant dyspnea management in this opioid-naïve patient.

References

1. Bruera E, Macmillan K, Pither J, MacDonald RN. Effects of morphine on the dyspnea of terminal cancer patients. *J Pain Symptom Manage*. 1990;5(6):341–344.
2. Kamal AH, Maguire JM, Wheeler JL, Currow DC, Abernethy AP. Dyspnea review for the palliative care professional: treatment goals and therapeutic options. *J Palliat Med*. 2012;15(1):106–114.
3. Jennings AL, Davies AN, Higgins JP, Gibbs JS, Broadley KE. A systematic review of the use of opioids in the management of dyspnoea. *Thorax*. 2002;57(11):939–944.
4. Vargas-Bermudez A, Cardenal F, Porta-Sales J. Opioids for the management of dyspnea in cancer patients: evidence of the last 15 years—a systematic review. *J Pain Palliat Care Pharmacother*. 2015;29(4):341–352.
5. Cabezon-Gutierrez L, Khosravi-Shahi P, Custodio-Cabello S, Muniz-Gonzalez F, Cano-Aguirre Mdel P, Alonso-Viteri S. Opioids for management of episodic breathlessness or dyspnea in patients with advanced disease. *Support Care Cancer*. 2016;24(9):4045–4055.

17

Palliative Oxygen Versus Room Air for Refractory Dyspnea

JASON A. WEBB AND ARIF H. KAMAL

> This study shows that compared with room air delivered by a nasal cannula, oxygen provides no additional symptomatic benefit for relief of refractory breathlessness.
>
> —ABERNETHY ET AL.[1]

Research Question: Is oxygen effective for the palliation of dyspnea among patients with normal blood oxygen levels (PaO2 > 7.3kPa)?

Funding: US National Institutes of Health, Australian National Health and Medical Research Council, Duke Institute for Care at the End of Life, and Doris Duke Charitable Foundation.

Year Study Began: 2006.

Year Study Published: 2010.

Study Location: Outpatient pulmonary, palliative care, oncology, and primary care clinics at five sites in Australia, two in the United States, and two in the UK.

Who Was Studied: Adults age >18 years of age, with PaO2 > 7.3kPa (i.e. PaO2 > 55 mmHg, 88% oxygen [O2] saturation), refractory dyspnea related to a life-limiting illness (determined by a referring physicians), receiving maximal treatment for the underlying disease, reported dyspnea at rest or with minimal exertion (≤3 on Medical Research Council categorical dyspnea scale), on stable medications for 1 week before participation, and expected survival of ≥ 1 month.

Who Was Excluded: Patients who met international eligibility criteria for long-term oxygen therapy; had a history of hypercarbic respiratory failure with oxygen, anemia, hypercarbia, or cognitive impairment; smoked; or had had a respiratory or cardiac event in the past 7 days.

How Many Patients: 239.

Study Overview: This study was an international, multicenter, double-blind, randomized controlled trial (Figure 17.1).

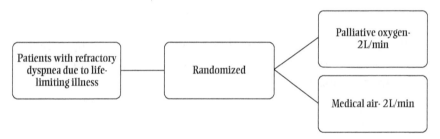

Figure 17.1 Summary of study design.

Study Intervention: Participants with refractory dyspnea due to life-limiting illness with PaO2 > 7.3kPa were randomly assigned in 1:1 ratio to receive oxygen or room air delivered by a concentrator and nasal cannula.

Palliative oxygen or medical air was administered continuously at 2L/min through nasal cannula. The concentrators for room air and oxygen were identical in appearance to all study participants. The intervention lasted for 7 days, and patients were instructed to use the concentrator for at least 15 hour/day.

Patients, individuals delivering the interventions, investigators, and nurses were masked to treatment assignments.

Follow-up: 7 days.

Endpoints: Primary outcome was "breathlessness right now," recorded by the patient twice daily (morning and evening) with a numeric rating scale from 0 to 10, with 10 = "breathlessness as bad as you can imagine."

RESULTS

- The primary outcome, breathlessness, did not differ between palliative oxygen and room air (Table 17.1).

Table 17.1. SUMMARY OF STUDY'S KEY FINDINGS[a]

	Oxygen Group (Absolute Change [95% CI]/ Relative Change [%])	Room Air Group (Absolute Change [95% CI]/ Relative Change [(%)])	Overall (Absolute Change [95% CI]/ Relative Change [%])	P Value
Change in AM Dyspnea	−0.9 (−1.3 to −0.5) −20%	−0.7 (−1.2 to −0.2) −15%	−0.8 (−1.1 to −0.5) −18%	0.504
Change in PM Dyspnea	−0.3 (−0.7 to 0.1) −7%	−0.5 (−0.9 to −0.1) −11%	−0.4 (−0.7 to −0.1) −9%	0.554
Change in Global QoL	0.7 (0.4 to 1.0) 11%	0.7 (0.4 to 1.0) 12%	0.7 (0.5 to 0.9) 12%	0.966

NOTE: CI = confidence interval; QoL = quality of life.

[a]Baseline to Day 6 using numeric rating scale.

- Morning dyspnea—52% (58/112 patients) responded to oxygen, and 40% (40/101 patients) responded to room air. Evening dyspnea— response rates were 42% for both interventions (oxygen, n = 47; room air, n = 42).
- Measures of quality of life did not differ between oxygen and room air.
- No significant adverse side effects were reported in either group, with no difference in extreme drowsiness reported.

Criticisms and Limitations:

- The primary outcome was dyspnea "now", which may be subjected to more fluctuations at the time of assessment, contributing to the negative findings. A more stable outcome for this study spanning multiple days may be average dyspnea over last 24 hours.
- The study population is primarily Caucasian males with advanced chronic obstructive pulmonary disease (COPD) and lung cancer, limiting the generalizability of the findings.

- The study findings cannot be extrapolated to patients in the last weeks of life as the study excluded patients with a prognosis of <1 month.

Other Relevant Studies and Information:

- A systematic review and meta-analysis of oxygen therapy for relief of dyspnea in patients with COPD found a modest reduction in dyspnea when compared to medical air (SMD = –0.3 (95% confidence interval [CI] –0.50 to –0.24; I^2 = 14%).[2] The discrepancy between the results of this review and the Abernethy trial may be due to the inclusion of patients with advanced cancer in the Abernathy trial. Uronis et al. demonstrated in a systematic review and meta-analysis that for cancer patients with dyspnea who are mildly or non-hypoxemic, oxygen failed to improve dyspnea (SMD = - 0.09, 95% CI –0.22 to 0.04; P = 0.16).[3]
- A randomized trial by Gailbraith et al. demonstrated that a handheld fan directed to the face significantly (P = 0.003) reduced the sensation of breathlessness for patients with life-limiting illnesses. Handheld fans can be inexpensive, are portable, enhance self-efficacy, and are widely available.[4]

Summary and Implications: This large international, multi-center, randomized controlled trial demonstrated no clinically significant symptomatic benefit of palliative oxygen versus room air delivered via nasal cannula for 7 days in patients with life-limiting illnesses and refractory dyspnea. Other studies have demonstrated a modest benefit of oxygen therapy for managing symptoms of dyspnea among patients with COPD, however.

CLINICAL CASE: SHOULD THIS PATIENT WITH BREATHLESSNESS BE TREATED WITH PALLIATIVE OXYGEN?

Case History

A 57-year-old man with stage IV metastatic adenocarcinoma of the lung presents to palliative care clinic for new consultation for symptom management. He reports dyspnea at rest and with minimal exertion for the past 6 weeks. He is on optimal therapy with bronchodilators, corticosteroids, low-dose oral morphine, and smoking cessation. He had a 6-minute walk test at his last pulmonary visit with an ambulatory oxygen saturation of 90% on room air.

He inquires as to whether he can get home oxygen for his breathlessness.

Suggested Answer

The Abernethy trial evaluated the symptomatic benefit of palliative oxygen therapy delivered via nasal cannula for refractory dyspnea and found no difference with room air. Studies have examined alternative therapies for dyspnea in patients with advanced cancer and COPD with findings that a hand-held fan may be adequate to provide some symptomatic benefit with dyspnea. If the patient had demonstrated ambulatory hypoxia the benefit with oxygen would have been greater as compared to a non-hypoxic patient. Thus, based on the Abernethy trial, in this case scenario, one could recommend against oxygen therapy due to the lack of symptomatic benefit compared to room air and potentially the burden and safety risks of carrying a concentrator.

References

1. Abernethy AP, McDonald CF, Frith PA, et al. Effect of palliative oxygen versus room air in relief of breathlessness in patients with refractory dyspnoea: a double-blind, randomized controlled trial. *Lancet*. 2010 Sep 4;376 (9743):784–793.
2. Uronis HE, Ekström MP, Currow DC, et al. Oxygen for relief of dyspnea in people with chronic obstructive pulmonary disease who would not qualify for home oxygen: a systematic review and meta-analysis. *Thorax*. 2015;70:492–494.
3. Uronis HE, Currow DC, McCrory DC, et al. Oxygen relief of dyspnea in mildly or non-hypoxaemic patients with cancer: a systematic review and meta-analysis. *Br J Cancer*. 2008;98:294–299.
4. Galbraith S, Fagan P, Perkins, P, et al. Does the use of a handheld fan improve chronic dyspnea? A randomized, controlled, crossover trial. *J Pain Symptom Manage*. 2010 May;39(5):831–838.

18

Exercise for the Management of Cancer-Related Fatigue

LYNN A. FLINT AND ERIC WIDERA

> Aerobic exercise can be regarded as beneficial for individuals with cancer-related fatigue during and post-cancer therapy, specifically for those with solid tumors.
>
> —Cramp and Byron-Daniel[1]

Research Question: Is exercise an effective treatment for cancer-related fatigue?

Funding: Faculty of Health and Social Care, University of the West of England, UK, and National Institute for Health Research Health Technology Assessment Programme, UK.

Year Study Began: 2007.

Year Study Published: 2012, updated from original 2008 review.

Study Location: Not applicable.

Who Was Studied: Cancer patients. The review included randomized, controlled trials evaluating exercise interventions in adults with cancer of any type and stage, at any point during or after treatment.

Who Was Excluded:

- Studies evaluating exercise as part of a larger intervention composed of multiple components were excluded because the effects of exercise alone could not be identified.
- The authors also excluded studies that did not provide details about the intervention, such as exercise type, duration, or frequency.
- Studies where the intervention consisted of only education or advice about exercise were excluded.
- Studies that did not report posttest means and those lacking a control arm were excluded from meta-analysis. These studies were included in the systematic review if they met other inclusion and exclusion criteria.

How Many Patients: This review included 56 studies.

Study Overview:

- The authors conducted a systematic review and meta-analysis of randomized-controlled trials that investigated the effect of exercise on cancer-related fatigue in adults during and after treatment (Figure 18.1).

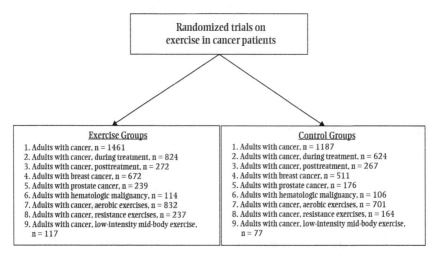

Figure 18.1 Summary of study design.

- The authors analyzed the studies as a whole group and as subgroups according to treatment phase, type of cancer, and type of exercise.

Study Intervention: Aerobic and resistance exercises.

Follow-up: Not applicable.

Endpoints: The primary outcome of the meta-analyses was patient report of fatigue using a variety of measures. The systematic review reported on anxiety, depression, quality of life, aerobic capacity, time spent exercising, and self-efficacy for ability to maintain physical activity and exercise maintenance on follow-up.

RESULTS

- 56 studies in total were included in the review (Figure 18.2).

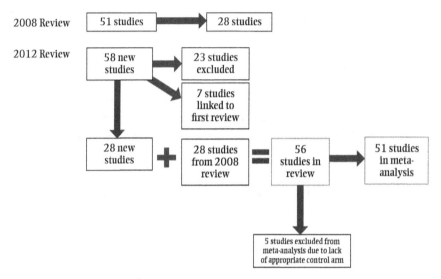

Figure 18.2 Included Studies.

- Meta-analyses
  - In the analysis of all studies, exercise was associated with statistically significant improvements in cancer-related fatigue as compared with control.
  - The subgroup analyses indicated that exercise was associated with statistically significant improvements in cancer-related fatigue in patients with breast and prostate cancer. No difference was found for patients with other types of cancer.
  - A subgroup analysis of exercise type showed that aerobic exercise, but not strength training or mind-body exercise, was associated with a statistically significant improvement in cancer-related fatigue.
  - A nonsignificant trend favoring exercise was found in studies limited to patients with hematologic malignancies.

- Resistance exercise and mind-body exercise also were associated with a trend toward improved fatigue.
- Systematic review
  - 19 of the 35 studies measuring quality of life showed a significant improvement on at least one quality of life instrument with exercise.
  - 15 of the 32 studies investigating aerobic capacity showed a significant improvement with exercise.
  - 13 of the 19 studies measuring anxiety showed no significant difference between intervention and control groups.
  - 19 of the 28 studies measuring depression found no significant difference between intervention and control groups.
  - A single study measuring exercise self-efficacy found no difference with an exercise intervention.

Criticisms and Limitations:

- The majority of included studies had small sample sizes.
- Few studies included patients with incurable cancer and/or poor performance status, limiting generalizability. Fatigue is particularly common in these individuals and can be debilitating.
- The included studies were clinically diverse in terms of patient characteristics and diagnoses, interventions, and concurrent treatments.
- There was at least a moderate degree of heterogeneity, or variation in study outcomes between studies, for each comparison including the overall comparison of exercise versus control for all adults with cancer.
- Included studies used a variety of different tools to measuring fatigue, limiting the ability to make direct comparisons.
- Data may have been biased toward positive outcomes because the studies were not blinded. Publication bias may also have led to overestimation of the beneficial effects of exercise.
- Many of the individual studies did not provide details about patients who declined to participate.
- A majority of the studies focused on patients with breast cancer.
- Participants were susceptible to altering their behavior because they were being observed (Hawthorne Effect), limiting generalizability to "real-life" situations.

Other Relevant Studies and Information:

- A recent Cochrane Review of studies of exercise interventions for patients with breast cancer receiving adjuvant therapy showed a slight improvement in fatigue, improvement in physical fitness, and minimal to no difference in quality of life or mood.[3]

- A recent meta-analysis focused on aerobic exercise interventions of adults with cancer at any stage and cancer-related fatigue showed an improvement compared to control groups.[4]
- In a randomized, controlled trial of tai chi in patients receiving chemotherapy for lung cancer, intervention patients reported smaller increases in fatigue at 6 and 12 weeks into therapy from baseline than control patients.[5]
- A meta-analysis of 9 trials of exercise interventions in patients with acute leukemia showed no significant difference in reported fatigue.[6]
- The American Society of Clinical Oncology guideline for screening, assessment, and management of cancer-related fatigue recommends at least 150 minutes of aerobic exercise plus resistance training.[2]

Summary and Implications: Exercise is associated with improvement in cancer-related fatigue in adults with solid tumors during and after cancer treatment. The evidence is strongest for patients with breast and prostate cancer and for aerobic exercise interventions. More studies are needed to determine if other forms of exercise, such as resistance training and mind-body exercise, are effective for cancer-related fatigue. Given the low risk of exercise for most patients, it is a reasonable first-line treatment for cancer-related fatigue for those who can tolerate it.

CLINICAL CASE: WHAT KIND OF EXERCISE IS HELPFUL FOR CANCER-RELATED FATIGUE?

Case History

A 63-year-old woman is being treated for metastatic breast cancer with chemotherapy. She has had significant cancer-related fatigue that limits her daily activities. Based on the Cochrane Review, should her palliative care provider recommend exercise to improve the fatigue? What type of exercise should the provider recommend?

Suggested Answer

According to the review, aerobic exercise was associated with improvements in cancer-related fatigue for patients with solid tumors at any point in therapy. The studies reviewed did not provide enough data to support one type of aerobic exercise program over another (i.e., supervised vs. individual). The review did not include many studies including patients with advanced disease, limiting generalizability to this particular patient. The provider should work with the interprofessional team, the patient, and her family to determine whether an exercise program would be appropriate and, if so, what type of aerobic exercise program might work best for her.

References

1. Cramp F, Byron-Daniel J. Exercise for the management of cancer-related fatigue in adults. *Cochrane Database Syst Rev.* 2012;11.
2. Bower JE, Bak K, Berger A, et al. Screening, assessment, and management of fatigue in adult survivors of cancer: an American Society of Clinical oncology clinical practice guideline adaptation. *J Clin Oncol.* 2014;32:1840–1850.
3. Furmaniak AC, Menig M, Markes MH. Exercise for women receiving adjuvant therapy for breast cancer. *Cochrane Database Syst Rev.* 2016;9.
4. Tian, L, Lu HJ, Lin L, Hu Y. Effects of aerobic exercise on cancer-related fatigue: a meta-analysis of randomized controlled trials. *Support Care Cancer.* 2016;24:969–983.
5. Zhang LL, Wang SZ, Chen HL, Yuan AZ. Tai chi exercise for cancer-related fatigue in patients with lung cancer undergoing chemotherapy: a randomized controlled trial. *J Pain Symptom Manage.* 2016;51:501–511.
6. Zhou Y, Zhu J, Gu Z, Yin X. Efficacy of exercise interventions in patients with acute leukemia: a meta-analysis. *PLoS One.* 2016;11.

19

Reduction of Cancer-Related Fatigue with Dexamethasone

A Double-Blind, Randomized, Placebo-Controlled Trial in Patients with Advanced Cancer

CHIRAG A. PATEL

> Dexamethasone is more effective than placebo in improving cancer-related fatigue and quality of life in patients with advanced cancer.
> —Yennu et al.[1]

Research Question: Is dexamethasone more effective than placebo in reducing cancer-related fatigue (CRF) in patients with advanced cancer?

Funding: Mentored Research Scholar Grant from the American Cancer Society.

Year Study Began: 2006.

Year Study Published: 2013.

Study Location: Outpatient clinics of MD Anderson Cancer Center, Houston, TX; Lyndon B Johnson General Hospital, Houston, TX; and Four Seasons Hospice, Flat Rock, NC.

Who Was Studied: Patients with advanced cancer with ≥3 CRF-related symptoms rated ≥4 out of 10 on the Edmonton Symptom Assessment Scale (ESAS) (i.e., pain, fatigue, chronic nausea and anorexia/cachexia, sleep, depression, poor appetite).

Who Was Excluded: Patients with dexamethasone allergy, inability to complete baseline assessment forms, recent or current megestrol or corticosteroid use, anemia, history of HIV or diabetes, neutropenia, recent surgery, or ongoing infection.

How Many Patients: 132.

Study Overview: This was a double-blinded, randomized, placebo-controlled trial in which 132 patients were randomized to receive either placebo orally twice per day or dexamethasone 4mg orally twice per day for 14 days (Figure 19.1).

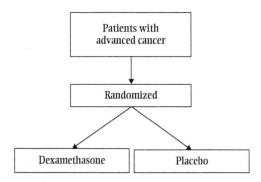

Figure 19.1 Summary of study design.

Study Intervention: Patients received either dexamethasone 4mg orally twice daily for 14 days or placebo orally twice daily for 14 days. A research nurse collected demographic and clinical data and supervised patients as they completed symptom assessment questionnaires at the time of random assignment. Assessments included Functional Assessment of Chronic Illness Therapy–Fatigue (FACIT-F), ESAS, Hospital Anxiety and Depression Scale (HADS), and Functional Assessment of Cancer Therapy–Anorexia–Cachexia (FAACT).

Follow-up: Questionnaires were again completed by patients on Days 8 and 15.

Endpoints: Primary outcome: Change in FACIT-F subscale from baseline to Day 15. Secondary outcomes: Change in anorexia (FAACT), anxiety and depression (HADS), and symptom distress scores (ESAS).

RESULTS

- 212 patients were assessed for eligibility, and 132 patients were randomly assigned: 65 patients were allocated to placebo and 67 patients were allocated to dexamethasone. By the end of the study, 84 patients were evaluable (41 patients in the placebo arm and 43 patients in the dexamethasone arm) (Table 19.1).

Table 19.1. SUMMARY OF STUDY'S KEY FINDINGS

| | Change in Symptom Scores (Mean ± SD) and P Value | | | | | |
| | Dexamethasone | Placebo | P Value | Dexamethasone | Placebo | P Value |
	15 Days	15 Days		8 Days	8 Days	
FACIT-F	9.0 ± 10.30	3.1 ± 9.59	0.008	8.01 ± 7.81	3.06 ± 7.28	0.005
FAACT	6.82 ± 8.95	1.95 ± 8.54	0.013	4.78 ± 8.44	1.49 ± 8.23	0.08
HADS Anxiety	−0.66 ± 3.45	−1.00 ± 3.54	0.75	−0.85 ± 3.16	−1.09 ± 2.32	0.59
HADS Depression	−1.39 ± 3.59	−0.31 ± 3.90	0.29	−1.23 ± 4.02	0.43 ± 3.12	0.65
ESAS Psychological SDS	−1.48 ± 4.67	−2.08 ± 4.73	0.65	−1.26 ± 4.68	−1.81 ± 5.01	0.65
ESAS Physical SDS	−10.68 ± 9.55	−4.78 ± 10.86	0.013	−9.10 ± 7.50	−3.42 ± 10.79	0.009

NOTE: FACIT-F = Functional Assessment of Chronic Illness Therapy–Fatigue; FAACT = Functional Assessment of Cancer Therapy–Anorexia–Cachexia; HADS = Hospital Anxiety and Depression Scale; SDS = Symptom Distress Score; ESAS = Edmonton Symptom Assessment Scale.

- FACIT-F subscale scores at Day 15 (primary outcome) and Day 8 showed significantly better mean improvement in the dexamethasone group compared to the placebo group.
- Anorexia scores (FAACT) improved significantly more in the dexamethasone group than placebo group at Day 15.
- Psychological symptoms were not improved more in the dexamethasone group compared to the placebo group. Improvement of HADS anxiety, HADS depression, FACIT-F emotional well-being, and ESAS psychological were not significantly improved in the dexamethasone group.
- Physical symptom scores improved more in the dexamethasone group than the placebo group. FACIT-F physical well-being and ESAS physical distress scores improved significantly more in the dexamethasone group then in the placebo group at Day 15.

Criticisms and Limitations:

- This study measured the effect of dexamethasone only until Day 15. Longer term efficacy and safety outcomes are not known.

- Only one dose (4mg twice daily) of dexamethasone therapy was examined.
- The inclusion criteria selected patients with symptom clusters instead of fatigue specifically, making it challenging to apply the findings in "real-world" clinical practice.

Other Relevant Studies and Information:

- The National Cancer Comprehensive Network Guidelines recommend consideration of steroids for short-term management of cancer-related fatigue among patients who are terminally ill or who have other concomitant indications (anorexia or pain related to brain/bone metastases).[2]

Summary and Implications: This prospective, placebo-controlled, randomized controlled trial of dexamethasone 4mg orally twice daily among patients with advanced cancer showed a reduction in CRF without an increase in significant adverse side effects relative to placebo at Days 8 and 15. Based on this and other studies, the National Cancer Comprehensive Network Guidelines recommends consideration of steroids for short-term management of cancer-related fatigue among patients who are terminally ill.

CLINICAL CASE: WHO SHOULD BE PRESCRIBED STEROIDS FOR CANCER-RELATED FATIGUE?

Case History

A 60-year-old female with right upper lobe lung cancer metastatic to liver and brain presents to an outpatient palliative care clinic with severe fatigue. She was referred from her oncologist, with whom she met earlier in the day. They discussed meeting with home hospice providers in the coming days given her preference to avoid further cancer-directed treatments due to fear of adverse side effects and progressive cancer despite first-line cytotoxic combination chemotherapy. She also describes moderate nausea and moderate anorexia.

Might this patient benefit from the palliative use of dexamethasone?

Suggested Answer

The Yennurajalingam trial evaluated the effects of dexamethasone and placebo on CRF for two weeks and found a significant improvement in fatigue levels in patients prescribed dexamethasone 4mg orally twice daily.

The patient in this case scenario could benefit from a course of dexamethasone, at least for short-term use, to ameliorate her cancer-related fatigue. Steroids may also improve her symptoms of nausea and anorexia.[3]

CRF is a multidimensional syndrome consisting of a "subjective sense of physical, emotional and/or cognitive tiredness or exhaustion related to cancer or cancer treatment that is not proportional to recent activity and interferes with usual functioning."[2] In addition to symptomatic treatment via corticosteroids or psychostimulants, a comprehensive approach to management of CRF in palliative care patients includes screening for and treatment of concurrent symptoms, evaluation for fatigue-inducing comorbidities, review of current medication profile, and education on self-management of fatigue.[4]

References

1. Yennurajalingam S, Frisbee-Hume S, Palmer JL. Reduction of cancer-related fatigue with dexamethasone: a double-blind, randomized, placebo-controlled trial in patients with advanced cancer. *J Clin Oncol.* 2013 Sept 1;31(25):3076–3082.
2. Berger A, Mooney K, Alvarez-Perez A, et al. Cancer-related fatigue, version 2. *J Natl Compr Canc Netw.* 2015 Aug;13(8):1012–1039.
3. Mercadante S, Fulfaro F, Casuccio A. The use of corticosteroids in home palliative care. *Support Care Cancer.* 2001 Jul;9(5):386–389.
4. de Raaf and van der Rijt: Can you help me feel less exhausted all the time? *J Clin Oncol.* 2013 Sept 1;31(25):3056–3060.

Parenteral Hydration in Patients with Advanced Cancer

CARLOS EDUARDO PAIVA AND
BIANCA SAKAMOTO RIBEIRO PAIVA

> This trial shows no benefits of parenteral hydration in end-of-life cancer patients no longer able to maintain adequate fluid intake.
>
> —BRUERA ET AL.[1]

Research Question: Does parenteral hydration improve symptoms associated with dehydration, delay the onset and/or severity of delirium, and affect the quality of life and survival in patients with advanced cancer no longer able to maintain adequate fluid intake?

Funding: National Cancer Institute and the M. D. Anderson Cancer Center Support Grant.

Year Study Began: 2007.

Year Study Published: 2013.

Study Location: 5 hospices from the Greater Houston, TX, area.

Who Was Studied: Adults with advanced cancers, admitted to hospice, with a reduced oral intake of fluids and with evidence of mild or moderate dehydration, reporting an intensity of ≥1 on a 0 to 10 scale for fatigue and two of the three other target symptoms (hallucinations, sedation, and myoclonus), life expectancy ≥1 week, availability of a primary caregiver, a Memorial Delirium Assessment Scale (MDAS) score less than 13, and ability to give written informed consent, living within 60 miles of the University of Texas MD Anderson Cancer Center.

Who Was Excluded: Patients with severe dehydration, a history or clinical evidence of congestive heart failure, or a history of bleeding disorders.

How Many Patients: 129.

Study Overview: This was a randomized, placebo-controlled, double-blind, multicenter study, in which patients with advanced cancer no longer able to maintain adequate fluid intake were randomized in a 1:1 ratio to receive parenteral hydration or a control (Figure 20.1).

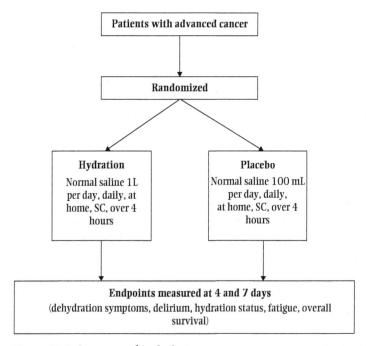

Figure 20.1 Summary of study design.

Study Intervention: Patients in the intervention group received 1 L of normal saline over 4 hours subcutaneously at home daily. Patients in the control group received 100 mL of normal saline over 4 hours daily. Patients were treated until they became unresponsive, developed progressive coma, or died. Both the patient and research nurse conducting the study assessments were blinded to the nature of the intervention.

Follow-up: 7 days.

Endpoints: Primary outcome: a change in the sum of four dehydration symptoms (fatigue, myoclonus, sedation, and hallucinations) between baseline and Day 4. Secondary outcome measures included delirium (MDAS, Richmond Agitation Sedation Scale [RASS], Nursing Delirium Screening Scale [NuDESC]), changes in the sum of four dehydration symptoms (fatigue, myoclonus, sedation, and hallucinations) between Day 7 and baseline, global symptom evaluation, quality of life using Functional Assessment of Chronic Illness Therapy–Fatigue (FACIT-F) and Functional Assessment of Chronic Illness Therapy–General (FACIT-G), hydration status using a dehydration assessment scale, laboratory data such as creatinine and blood urea nitrogen (BUN), and overall survival.

RESULTS

- There were improvements observed in the symptom profile and quality of life scores as well as delirium scores (MDAS and RASS) between baseline and Days 4 and 7 in both the hydration and control groups. The dehydration assessment scale scores improved from baseline in both the hydration and control groups at Day 4 but not Day 7 (Table 20.1).

Table 20.1. SUMMARY OF STUDY'S KEY FINDINGS

Outcomes	Change Between Day 4 and Baseline			Change Between Day 7 and Baseline		
	Hydration (Mean Δ)	Control (Mean Δ)	P Value	Hydration (Mean Δ)	Control (Mean Δ)	P Value
Sum of dehydration symptoms	–3.3[a]	–2.8[a]	0.77	–4.9	–3.8	0.54
RASS	0[a]	0[a]	0.07	0[a]	–1[a]	0.35
MDAS	1[a]	3.5[a]	0.08	2[a]	2.5[a]	0.44
NuDESC, night	0	0[a]	0.03	0	0	0.79
FACT-G	—	—	—	6.7[a]	2.6	0.31
FACT-F				9.1[a]	1.4	0.23
Dehydration scale	–0.8[a]	–0.6[a]	0.38	–1.0	–0.5[a]	0.13
BUN	—	—	—	–2	2	0.02

NOTE: RASS = Richmond Agitation Sedation Scale; MDAS = Memorial Delirium Assessment Scale; NuDESC = Nursing Delirium Screening Scale; FACIT-G = Functional Assessment of Chronic Illness Therapy–General; FACIT-F = Functional Assessment of Chronic Illness Therapy–Fatigue; BUN = blood urea nitrogen.

[a]P value < 0.05 (before-and-after analysis).

- No differences in primary and secondary outcomes were observed between study arms (hydration vs. control). The only exceptions were the secondary outcomes nighttime NuDESC (Day 4, control group showed significantly more deterioration from baseline compared with the hydration group) and BUN levels (Day 7, the hydration group had a significantly lower BUN level, which was not observed in the control group).
- The overall median survival was 17 days; there was no significant difference in median survival between the hydration and control groups (21 vs. 15 days; P = 0.83).

Criticisms and Limitations:

- The planned sample size (n = 150) was not achieved. Because of funding issues, the study was terminated after 129 patients.
- Patients with severe dehydration were excluded from this study, and thus the results may not apply to this population.
- Patients may take fluids by mouth. This co-intervention may reduce the potential benefit of parenteral hydration.

Other Relevant Studies and Information:

- A qualitative study that examined the meaning of hydration for terminally ill cancer patients in home hospice care and for their primary caregivers determined that they viewed fluids as enhancing comfort, dignity, and quality of life.[2]
- An update of a Cochrane Systematic Review published in 2014[3] that included the study by Bruera et al.[1] was conducted to evaluate the impact of hydration on the quality and length of life of palliative care patients. Only 6 studies were found; the small number of studies and their heterogeneity made it difficult to perform a meta-analysis. Taken together, the studies published did not show a significant benefit regarding the use of hydration in palliative care patients.
- A secondary analysis of the data focusing on the clinical utility of the NuDESC was published in subsequent article.[4] The NuDESC was not a reliable tool for screening for delirium when scoring was conducted by a caregiver (nighttime NuDESC), raising questions about the significance of the reduce nighttime delirium with IV hydration identified in this study.

Summary and Implications: This well-designed randomized controlled trial provides the highest level of evidence to date on the role of parenteral hydration in patients with weeks of life expectancy. Specifically, for patients with advanced cancer who are mildly to moderately dehydrated, parenteral hydration did not improve symptoms associated with dehydration, quality of life, or survival compared with standard oral hydration alone.

CLINICAL CASE: ARE THERE BENEFITS TO ROUTINE PARENTERAL HYDRATION AT END OF LIFE?

Case History

A 55-year-old man with advanced pancreatic cancer with metastasis to the liver and lung, with disease progression after two sequential lines of chemotherapy, is admitted to an acute palliative care unit. The Palliative Performance Score is 30%, and he has an estimate of 2 to 4 weeks of survival. He is no longer able to swallow solids, and his oral intake is also very limited. His family is very distressed and questions the need for parenteral hydration. The palliative care doctor discusses with the medical residents the actual indication of such a procedure in the context of mild to moderate dehydration and absence of hemodynamic abnormalities. What is the evidence for the benefits of parenteral hydration in this clinical setting?

Suggested Answer

The low fluid intake is a consequence of the natural progression of neoplasia. Although parenteral hydration is a common practice in hospitals, the benefit is less clear. The Bruera trial comparing subcutaneous daily parenteral hydration versus control in patients with mild to moderate dehydration did not show benefits in reducing symptoms related to dehydration, delirium diagnosis, quality of life scores, or improvement in overall survival. Thus our recommendation is that patients in a similar situation simply take sips of fluid as tolerated. However, given the relatively low risk of adverse effects as shown here, parenteral hydration is not unreasonable as a therapeutic trial if the family insisted.

References

1. Bruera E, Hui D, Dalal S, et al. Parenteral hydration in patients with advanced cancer: a multicenter, double-blind, control-controlled randomized trial. *J Clin Oncol.* 2013;31(1):111–118. doi:10.1200/JCO.2012.44.6518
2. Cohen MZ, Torres-Vigil I, Burbach BE, de la Rosa A, Bruera E. The meaning of parenteral hydration to family caregivers and patients with advanced cancer

receiving hospice care. *J Pain Symptom Manage.* 2012;43(5):855–865. doi:10.1016/ j.jpainsymman.2011.06.016

3. Good P, Richard R, Syrmis W, Jenkins-Marsh S, Stephens J. Medically assisted hydration for adult palliative care patients. In: Good P, ed. *Cochrane Database of Systematic Reviews.* Chichester, UK: John Wiley; 2014. doi:10.1002/14651858.CD006273. pub3

4. De la Cruz M, Noguera A, San Miguel-Arregui MT, Williams J, Chisholm G, Bruera E. Delirium, agitation, and symptom distress within the final seven days of life among cancer patients receiving hospice care. *Palliat Support Care.* 2015;13(02):211–216. doi:10.1017/S1478951513001144

21

Enteral Tube Feeding Dysphagic Stroke Patients

FRANCISCO LOAICIGA AND RONY DEV

> Early tube feeding might reduce case fatality, but at the expense of increasing the proportion surviving with poor outcome.
> —FOOD TRIAL COLLABORATION[1]

Research Question: Does the timing or route of enteral feeding affect clinical outcomes for patients with dysphagia following stroke? Specifically: (1) Is early or late enteral feeding preferable following stroke? and (2) Is nasogastric (NG) or percutaneous endoscopic gastrostomy (PEG) feeding the preferred route?

Funding: Health Technology Assessment Board of National Health Service Research and Development (UK), Stroke Association, Chief Scientist Office of the Scottish Executive, and Chest, Heart and Stroke Scotland.

Year Study Began: 1996.

Year Study Published: 2005.

Study Location: 15 countries across the globe (Australia, Belgium, Brazil, Canada, Czech Republic, Denmark, Hong Kong, India, Italy, New Zealand, Portugal, Republic of Ireland, Singapore, UK).

Who Was Studied: The study enrolled any patient hospitalized with a recent (within 7 days before admission) stroke (first-ever or recurrent) if the responsible clinician was uncertain of the best feeding policy.

Who Was Excluded: Patients with subarachnoid hemorrhage.

How Many Patients: 859 patients in the analysis examining the timing of feeding and 321 patients in the analysis comparing PEG insertion versus NG feeding.

Study Overview: The first study compared early feeding versus avoiding nutrition (Figure 21.1).

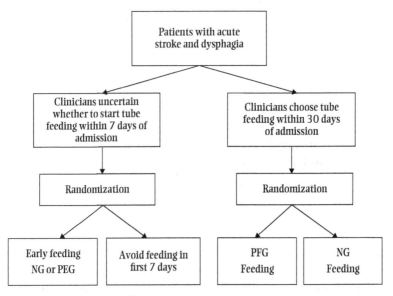

Figure 21.1 Summary of study design.

- Arm 1: Early feeding—Patients with dysphagia following stroke were allocated early enteral nutrition via mixed NG and PEG.
- Arm 2: Delayed feeding—Patients with dysphagia following stroke were allocated to avoid tube feedings for at least 7 days.

The second study compared PEG versus NG tube feeding in dysphagic patients after a stroke.

- Arm 1: PEG insertion—Dysphagic stroke patients received a PEG tube for enteral nutrition
- Arm 2: NG feeding—Dysphagic stroke patients allocated to placement of a nasogastric tube

Endpoints: Two primary endpoints were (1) death at 6 months and (2) death or poor outcome at 6 months. Patients with a modified Rankin Score of Grade 4 (moderately severe disability; unable to walk without assistance, and unable to attend to own bodily needs without assistance) or Grade 5 (severe disability; bedridden, incontinent, and requiring constant nursing care and attention) were considered to have poor outcome. Secondary outcomes included place of residence, quality of life score, compliance with treatment, length of hospital stay, in-hospital complications, and cause of death.

Follow-up: 6 months.

RESULTS

- Early versus delayed feeding analysis (Table 21.1):

Table 21.1. SUMMARY OF STUDY's KEY FINDINGS

MRS	Early Tube Feeding (n = 429)	Delayed Tube Feeding (n = 430)	PEG Tube Feeding (n = 162)	Nasogastric Tube Feeding (n = 159)
Dead	182 (42%)	207 (48%)	79 (49%)	76 (48%)
MRS 0–3 (good outcome)	90 (21%)	85 (20%)	18 (11%)	30 (19%)
MRS 4–5 (poor outcome)	157 (37%)	137 (32%)	65 (40%)	53 (33%)
Dead or MRS 4–5	339 (79%)	344 (80%)	144 (89%)	129 (81%)

NOTE: MRS = Modified Rankin Scale; PEG = percutaneous endoscopic gastrostomy.

- There was no difference between arms with respect to death or poor outcomes at 6 months; however, there was a nonstatistically significant trend favoring the early feeding arm for the risk the death (absolute risk reduction 5.8% (95% confidence interval [CI] –0.8 to 12.5%, P = 0.09) and the risk of death or poor outcome (absolute risk reduction 1.2% (95% CI –4.2 to 6.6; P = 0.7).
- No significant differences were reported between groups in the secondary outcomes, including the frequency of recurrent strokes, pneumonia, urinary infections, or venous thromboembolism. However, the rate of gastrointestinal hemorrhage was higher with early versus delayed feeding (22 vs. 11 patients, P = 0.04).
- PEG versus enteral trial:
  - Percutaneous endoscopic gastrostomy feeding was associated with a nonsignificant increase in the risk of death of 1.0% (–10.0% to 11.9%,

P = 0.9) and a borderline significant increase in the risk of death or poor outcome 7.8% (0.0% to 15.5%, P = 0.05).
- NG was associated with a higher rate of gastrointestinal hemorrhage compared to PEG (18 vs. 5 patients, P = 0.005). No significant differences were reported between groups regarding the frequency of recurrent strokes, pneumonia, urinary infections, or venous thromboembolism.

Criticisms and Limitations:

- This study was terminated early because of funding issues. The investigators were only able to recruit 859 of 2,000 planned patients for the early/avoid trial and 321 of 1,000 planned patients in the PEG/enteral trial. Thus it is underpowered to detect a statistical difference in the various outcomes.
- A small proportion of patients crossed over to the other study arms, which could decrease the treatment effect.
- The assessment of poor outcome was done by mail questionnaire or telephone interview 6 months after the enrollment in the study instead of an in-person interview.
- Patients were enrolled if clinicians were uncertain whether to start tubefeeding or which type of tubefeeding should be provided when the study was being conducted. However, publication of study findings may shift the clinicians' understanding of the risk/benefits ratio. Thus it may not be possible to identify patients who met the "same study eligibility criteria" to apply the study findings.

Other Relevant Studies and Information:

- A recent Cochrane Review of randomized controlled trials compared timing and route (PEG vs. NG) of tube feeding.[2] The reviewers identified 33 studies involving 6,779 patients reported no survival difference between PEG and NG tubefeeds, but PEG feeding was associated with elevated albumin concentration, higher caloric intake, and less complications of gastrointestinal bleeding. In addition, no difference in mortality or dependency was noted with early versus late initiation of tube feeding.

Summary and Implications: This large, multicenter trial represents the most ambitious effort to date to address some important questions regarding tubefeeding for patients with dysphagia following stroke. Early initiation of tube feeding (within 7 days of hospitalization) may be associated with a small survival benefit relative to delayed initiation; however, many of those who survived because of the early feeding intervention had poor functional outcomes. This analysis also demonstrated that NG tube may be preferred over PEG tube because of better outcomes, though it was underpowered to demonstrate this conclusively.

CLINICAL CASE: WOULD YOU RECOMMEND ENTERAL TUBE FEEDING FOR THIS PATIENT?

Case History

A 77-year-old male, with past medical history pertinent for coronary artery disease, hypertension, and hypercholesterolemia, was diagnosed with acute stroke with complications of residual hemiparesis and dysphagia.

A family member has noted decreased oral intake and is inquiring about PEG tube placement or NG tube placement.

Should you recommend PEG tube, NG tube, or none?

Suggested Answer

Patients and their caregivers should be informed that early tube feeding might reduce mortality but may result in their loved one surviving with worse functional outcomes. If early feeding is pursued, dysphagic stroke patients may be offered enteral feeding via a NG tube within the first few days of admission and is preferred over PEG feeding. A conversation should be held with patient and caregivers regarding benefits, limitations, and complications associated with various enteral feedings for stroke patients with dysphagia prior to initiation.

References

1. Food Trial Collaboration. Effect of timing and method of enteral tube feeding for dysphagic stroke patients (FOOD): a multicenter randomized controlled trial. *Lancet.* 2005;365:764–772.
2. Geeganage C, Beavan J, Ellender S, Bath PM. Interventions for dysphagia and nutritional support in acute and subacute stroke. *Cochrane Database Syst Rev.* 2012;10:CD000323.

22

Feeding Tube and Survival Among Patients with Severe Cognitive Impairment

CLAUDIO ADILE

> [For patients with severe cognitive impairment,] health care providers can have confidence that feeding tube does not prolong survival and that earlier timing of insertion does not affect survival, as well.
>
> —TENO ET AL.[1]

Research Question: Does feeding tube insertion and its timing improve survival?

Funding: National Institute of Aging Research.

Year Study Began: 1999 (starting date of the data set).

Year Study Published: 2012.

Study Location: US nursing homes.

Who Was Studied: All US nursing home residents with severe cognitive impairment and the need for eating assistance.

Who Was Excluded: Comatose patients, those who died within 2 weeks of assessment, and those with percutaneous endoscopic gastrostomy (PEG) feeding in the prior 6 months.

How Many Patients: 34,536.

Study Overview: See Figure 22.1 for a summary of the study design.

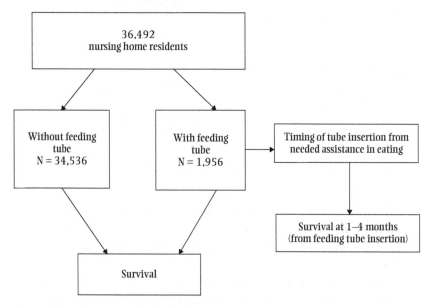

Figure 22.1 Summary of study design.

Study Intervention: Patients with feeding tube insertion versus no feeding tube insertion.

Follow-up: Not applicable.

Endpoints: Overall survival.

RESULTS

- Of the 36,492 nursing home residents (88.4% white, mean age 84.9, 87.4% with one feeding tube risk factor), 1,957 (5.4%) had a feeding tube inserted within 1 year of developing eating problems. African Americans and Hispanics were more likely to have a feeding tube inserted after the development of the need for assistance in eating. A greater percentage of residents without feeding tubes also had some documentation of advance care planning (i.e., living will, durable power of attorney for health care, do not resuscitate order) when compared to residents with feeding tubes (Table 22.1).

Table 22.1. ASSOCIATION BETWEEN THE PRESENCE AND TIMING OF
PEG TUBE INSERTION AND OVERALL SURVIVAL

	Adjusted Hazard Ratio (95% Confidence Interval)
Any PEG tube insertion	
Present	1.03 (0.94–1.13)
Absent	1 (reference)
Timing of PEG tube insertion	
In first month	1.01 (0.86–1.20)
In second month	1.12 (0.93–1.35)
In third month	0.82 (0.64–1.04)
In fourth month or later	1 (reference)

NOTE: PEG = percutaneous endoscopic gastrostomy.

- After multivariate analysis correcting for selection bias with propensity score weights, no difference was found in the survival in the two groups (adjusted hazard ratio 1.03, 95% confidence interval [CI] 0.94–1.13).
- Among residents who received a tube feeding, the timing of PEG tube insertion relative to the onset of eating problems was not associated with improved survival post feeding tube insertion (adjusted hazard ratio 1.01, 95% CI 0.86–1.20).

Criticisms and Limitations:

- Propensity score analysis can only account for some known variables. Some confounders are not included (e.g., patient preference for feeding tube and other life-prolonging measures). Randomized controlled trials may overcome this to a certain extent but are logistically more difficult to conduct.
- The study findings are limited to nursing home residents with cognitive impairment with a median survival of approximately 6 months.

Other Relevant Studies and Information:

- Prior research suggests that feeding tubes are not associated with improved survival. These studies, however, had some limitations, including using a single institution and including both nasogastric tubes and PEG tubes. Also, none of the studies used techniques to control for potential selection bias.[1,2]

- The American Geriatrics Society published a guideline in 2014 advising against the use of feeding tubes in older patients with advanced dementia because of the lack of proven benefit and increased risks such as agitation, tube-related complications, and pressure ulcers.[3]

Summary and Implications: This important study found that feeding tubes insertion does not confer a survival benefit among nursing home residents with severe cognitive impairment. Moreover, an earlier insertion of feeding tubes in this patient population is not associated with improved survival.

CLINICAL CASE: SHOULD THIS PATIENT RECEIVE A FEEDING TUBE?

Case History

Mr. Jefferson is a 79-year-old man with advanced dementia who is noncommunicative. He was brought to the emergency room from his nursing home due to needing assistance in eating, failure to thrive, and weight loss of 30 lbs over the past 3 months. His only daughter, who is also the medical power of attorney, believes he is no longer able to interact with her. She is wondering if a feeding tube should be inserted. What should guide the decision making regarding a feeding tube?

Suggested Answer

The disease trajectory of dementia includes substantial functional impairment, profound aphasia, loss of mobility, and the development of eating problems in the last year of life. Many would perceive this quality of life as poor and that the insertion of a feeding tube would merely prolong a dying process without a meaningful quality of life. Nonetheless, family members often cite survival as a principal reason for choosing to insert a feeding tube, particularly in patients who did not express their intention regarding end-of-life issues. Given the methodological rigor of this study, the physician can inform the daughter that feeding tube does not prolong survival in patients with advanced dementia. In fact, insertion of a feeding tube may result in potential complications and does not prevent aspiration.

References

1. Finucane TE, Christmas C, Travis K. Tube feeding in patients with advanced dementia: A review of the evidence. *JAMA*. 1999;282:1365–1370.
2. Gillick MR. Rethinking the role of tube feeding in patients with advanced dementia. *N Engl J Med*. 2000;342:206–210.
3. American Geriatrics Society feeding tubes in advanced dementia position statement. *J Am Geriatr Soc*. 2014;62(8):1590–1593.

23

Parenteral Nutrition in Cancer Patients Undergoing Chemotherapy

FRANCISCO LOAICIGA AND RONY DEV

> Routine use of TPN in patients undergoing chemotherapy should be strongly discouraged, and trials involving specific groups of patients or modifications in TPN should be undertaken with caution.
>
> —McGeer et al.[1]

Research Question: What is the effect of total parenteral nutrition (TPN) support on survival, tumor response, and toxicity in cancer patients undergoing chemotherapy?

Funding: National Center for Health Services Research, the Health Care Technology Assessment, and the National Health Research and Development Program (Canada).

Year Study Began: 1966–1986.

Year Study Published: 1990.

Study Location: 15 randomized controlled trials, including studies from the United States, Canada, and Europe.

Who Was Studied: 31 published reports were identified and 15 randomized controlled trials were included in meta-analysis. Included studies involved randomized controlled trials evaluating TPN as an adjunct to chemotherapy in adult and pediatric patients with various solid and hematological malignancies.

Who Was Excluded: 31 published reports were identified in the literature review process; 7 of these studies were rejected: 3 were uncontrolled, 1 tested central versus peripheral TPN, 2 provided no data to support the conclusions, and 1 study permitted multiple crossovers, blurring the distinction between the treatment groups.

How Many Patients: 293.

Study Overview: See Figure 23.1 for a summary of the study design.

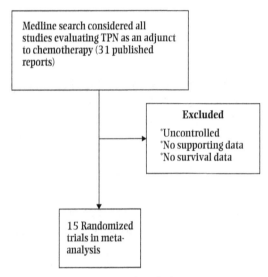

Figure 23.1 Summary of study design.

Study Intervention: All randomized controlled trials included evaluated TPN as an adjunct to chemotherapy.

Study Outcomes:

- Survival at 3 months and overall survival
- Tumor response rate (complete or partial) to chemotherapy
- Chemotherapy toxicity: infectious, hematologic, and gastrointestinal

- Number of major complications of TPN (rates of catheter-related sepsis, pneumothorax, symptomatic, venous thrombosis)
- Length of hospital stay

Follow-up: Not applicable.

RESULTS

- Survival: Overall, there was not statistically significant difference between TPN and no TPN. No individual study demonstrated a beneficial effect of TPN. When pooling the data, the reviewers concluded that TPN-treated patients were 80% as likely to survive versus patients in the control group. When only high-quality studies were considered, the size of the detrimental effect of TPN on survival increased (Table 23.1).

Table 23.1. Summary of Study's Key Findings

		Pooled Odds Ratio for TPN vs. No TPN (95% CI)	P Value
Overall survival	Baseline studies	0.81 (0.62–1.0)	0.06
3-month survival	Baseline studies	0.74 (0.42–1.3)	0.29
	Quality weighted	0.61 (0.23–1.6)	0.30
Tumor response	Baseline studies	0.68 (0.40–1.1)	0.12
	All studies	0.80 (0.50-1.3)	0.33
	Quality weighted	0.67 (0.28–1.6)	0.22
Risk of infection	Baseline studies	4.1 (2.4–6.9)	<0.001
	All studies	3.1 (1.9–5.0)	<0.005
	Quality weighted	4.2 (1.7–10.6)	<0.005

NOTE: TPN = total parenteral nutrition; CI = confidence interval.

- Tumor response: Overall, there was no statistically significant difference between TPN and no TPN. In the pooled data, a trend against TPN was noted with lower rates of complete and partial response to chemotherapy. When the reviewers evaluated only high-quality studies, the estimated detrimental effect of TPN increased. In patients with a complete response, a nonsignificant trend for a benefit for TPN was noted. Amount and timing of TPN, patient age, and concomitant radiotherapy had no impact on the benefit of TPN; however, there was a trend toward less detrimental effect of TPN in malnourished patients.

- Infection: The meta-analysis reported higher rates of infection in cancer patients receiving TPN, and increased infection risk persisted after the authors excluded catheter-related infections from the analysis.
- Length of hospital stay: The use of TPN resulted in prolongation of hospital stay by a median of 14 days.
- Hematologic and gastrointestinal toxicity and major complications: Data was too heterogeneous and not analyzed. The rates of major complications of TPN were similar to reported frequency in surgical patients.

Criticism and Limitations:

- Selection of trials to be included and outcomes may have introduced a bias in the final analysis, but the authors did follow a carefully designed and prespecified protocol.
- The validity of the authors' assessment of study quality has not been established.
- Infection criteria were unclear in many of the lower quality studies included in the meta-analysis.

Other Relevant Studies and Information:

- A review analyzing the emotional decisions faced by patients, caregivers, and health care providers on the use of parenteral nutrition in patients with advanced cancer[2] emphasized that parenteral nutrition should not become reactionary response to the fear of starvation and carries the burden of administrating parenteral nutrition bags, frequent blood draws, and noisy intravenous infusion pumps, which run continuously throughout the night.
- A prospective crossover controlled study of 43 cancer patients evaluating the effectiveness in TPN in improving nutritional status in cancer patients undergoing chemotherapy[3] found no difference in toxicity or improvement in nutritional status with administration of TPN.
- The 2016 European Society for Clinical Nutrition and Metabolism guideline on nutrition in cancer patients recommended the use of parenteral nutrition to maintain nutritional status in (1) patients undergoing curative anticancer therapies if enteral nutrition is insufficient or incompatible and (2) highly selected patients with advanced cancer with adequate prognosis and in whom parenteral

nutrition is expected to provide a significant benefit. The use of parenteral nutrition among patients in the terminal phase of cancer is not recommended.

Summary and Implications: In this groundbreaking meta-analysis, the routine use of TPN in patients with cancer undergoing chemotherapy was associated with increased risk of infections and a nonstatistically significant trend toward decreased survival and lower tumor response rate to chemotherapy. However, a subgroup of patients, such as those who were seriously malnourished and those with mechanical obstruction but otherwise good life expectancy, may derive some benefit from TPN. More research is needed to further elucidate this possibility.

CLINICAL CASE: PARENTERAL NUTRICION IN CANCER PATIENTS UNDERGOING CHEMOTHERAPY

Case History

A 56-year-old female patient with widely metastatic lung cancer on third-line palliative chemotherapy has significant weight loss over 30 lbs over the past 3 months, anorexia, and fatigue. She has an Eastern Cooperative Oncology Group scale performance status of 3. The patient's husband is inquiring about the possibility of TPN as a way to maintain nutritional status and "maybe regain strength to continue chemotherapy." What would you recommend for this patient?

Suggested Answer

This patient likely has less than 3 months of survival. TPN may be harmful to her, with a higher rate of infection and possibly lower likelihood of survival and treatment response. Thus TPN is not recommended. In fact, this is a good opportunity to have further goals of care discussions and to talk to the patient regarding whether or not chemotherapy is compatible with her goals.

References

1. McGreer AJ, Detsky AS, O'Rourke K. Parenteral nutrition in cancer patients undergoing chemotherapy: a meta-analysis. *Nutrition.* 1990;6(3):233–240.
2. Mitchell J, Jatoi A. Parenteral nutrition in patients with advanced cancer: merging perspectives from the patient and healthcare provider. *Semin Oncol.* 2011; 38(3):439–442.

3. De Cicco M, Panarello G, Fantin D, et. al. Parenteral nutrition in cancer patients receiving chemotherapy: effects on toxicity and nutritional status. *JPEN J Parenter Enteral Nutr* 1993;17(6):513–518.
4. Arends J, Bachmann P, Baracos V, et al. ESPEN guidelines on nutrition in cancer patients. *Clin Nutr.* 2017 Feb;36(1):11–48.

24

Docusate and Sennosides for Constipation

SHALINI DALAL

[D]ocusate plus sennosides was not more efficacious than sennosides alone in the management of constipation in hospice patients.

—TARUMI ET AL.[1]

Research Question: Is there a benefit of combining a stool softener, such as docusate, with a stimulant laxative, such as sennosides, in the management of constipation among hospice patients?

Funding: Funding agencies included

- College of Family Physicians of Canada (Janus Research Grant)
- Caritas Research Trust Fund
- Department of Family Medicine at the University of Alberta (summer studentship)
- Health Quality Council of Alberta (summer studentship)
- Alberta Innovates-Health Solutions (summer studentship)

Year Study Began: December 2005 to November 2010.

Year Study Published: 2013.

Study Location: 3 inpatient hospice units in Edmonton, Alberta.

Who Was Studied: Adult patients admitted to an inpatient hospice program with a Palliative Performance Scale status of 20% or greater.

Who Was Excluded: Patients with a gastrointestinal stoma tumor, contraindications to docusate, or recent use of docusate.

How Many Patients: 326 patients and 258 referring physicians.

Study Overview: This was a multicenter, randomized, double-blind, placebo-controlled trial (Figure 24.1).

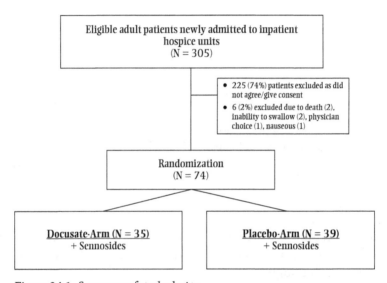

Figure 24.1 Summary of study design.

Study Intervention: Eligible hospice patients were randomly assigned to one of two groups, the docusate or placebo arm. The docusate group received two 100mg docusate (dioctyl sodium sulfosuccinate) tablets twice daily. Both arms received 1 to 3 sennoside tablets (8.6 mg/tablet) taken 1 to 3 times daily.

Endpoints:

Primary outcomes:
- Stool frequency as measured by patient self-report
- Stool volume as measured by patient self-report
- Stool consistency as measured by patient self-report

Secondary outcomes:

- Type and frequency of additional bowel care interventions
- Patient's perception of difficulty and completeness of evacuation
- Symptoms possibly related to constipation (pain, tiredness, nausea, drowsiness, anxiety, depression, appetite loss, well-being, and shortness of breath)

The study intervention was provided for 10 days. After that time, patients reverted back to their original bowel regimen.

RESULTS

- Overall, 75% patients completed the study: 25 (71%) in the docusate and 31 (80%) in the placebo arm. Reasons for noncompletion included the inability to swallow/discontinuation of oral medications (5 in each arm) and the team/family consensus to remove (2 each) (Table 24.1).
- Both groups received opioids during the study, with 92% to 94% of patients in the docusate arm and 100% in the placebo arm, during each of the 10 days of the trial.
- There was no significant difference in the mean morphine equivalent daily dosage between the docusate (93mg) and placebo (154mg; $P = 0.26$) arms.
- There was no significant difference in the primary outcome of the mean number of bowel movements (BM) per day between the two groups (Table 24.1).
- There was no significant difference between the proportion of patients who had a BM on 50% or more study days in the docusate and placebo arms (56% vs. 71%; $P = 0.44$) or in the proportion of patients who had at least one BM in 3 days (71% vs. 81%, $P = 0.45$).
- There was no significant difference in stool volumes between the two groups (large volume: 54% vs. 44%; $P = 0.06$).
- There was no significant difference in the need of ≥ 1 additional bowel care intervention between the placebo and docusate groups (74% vs. 69% patients; $P = 0.77$).
- There was no difference between the patients perception of BMs being difficult ($P = 0.57$) or for the sense of complete evacuation ($P = 0.77$).

Table 24.1. COMPARISON BETWEEN DOCUSATE PLACEBO GROUPS

Endpoints	Docusate	Placebo	P Value
Stool frequency			
• Mean number of BMs/day (SD)	0.74 (0.47)	0.69 (0.37)	0.58
• Patients with BM on 50% of days	56%	71%	0.44
• Patients with BM ≥ once every 3 days	71%	81%	0.45
Stool volume			
• Large volume	54%	44%	0.06
• Medium volume	30%	31%	
• Small volume	12%	21%	
Stool consistency (Bristol Stool Form Scale)	More patients with Type 3 (sausage, cracks in surface) and Type 6 (mushy stool, fluffy pieces with ragged edges) stool	More patients with Type 4 (smooth and soft, like a sausage or snake) and Type 5 (soft blobs with clear-cut edges) stool	0.01
Need for additional bowel care interventions (%)			
• Needed ≥1 intervention	69%	74%	0.77
• Needed intervention on Day 5	14%	39%	0.35
Patient's perception of BM			
• Difficult evacuation	33%	25%	0.57
• Sense of complete evacuation	74%	79%	0.77

NOTE: BM = bowel movement; SD = standard deviation.

Criticisms and Limitations:

- This small study was not powered for equivalency or noninferiority. Thus the lack of statistical significance cannot prove that the two study arms were equivalent.
- This study did not specifically enroll patients who were constipated, and so the study interventions were used more for preventative purposes.

Also, although they initially limited study entry to patients on opioids, this criterion was removed halfway through the study period to facilitate patient enrollment.
- Only a minority of eligible patients agreed to participate in this study, which may have generated a selection bias.

Other Relevant Studies and Information:

- A systematic review on docusate in chronically ill patients included 4 studies.[2] The investigators concluded that there was inadequate evidence to support its use and more research is necessary.
- A retrospective cohort study comparing senna plus docusate vs. senna also found that addition of docusate did not provide further benefit.[3]
- The most recent (2015) Cochrane Systematic Review[2] on laxatives for the management of constipation among patients receiving palliative care identified 5 studies and concluded there was no differences in the effectiveness between the different laxatives that were studied, including sennosides, docusate, lactulose, herbal compounds, otherapy sennosides/lactulose with magnesium hydroxide plus liquid paraffin.[4] However, more research is necessary given the paucity of clinical trials on this topic.
- Polyethylene glycol is frequently used in the management of constipation, but there are no trials of polyethylene glycol among palliative care patients. However, a systematic review in the nonpalliative population reported superiority of polyethylene glycol vs.lactulose.[5]

Summary and Implications: This study, one of the few randomized trials on constipation in the palliative care setting, addresses a commonly asked question in clinical practice. It found that adding docusate to therapy with sennosides is no more efficacious than sennosides alone among patients enrolled in hospice.

CLINICAL CASE: IS THERE A BENEFIT OF ADDING DOCUSATE TO SENNA IN THE MANAGEMENT OF CONSTIPATION IN THE PALLIATIVE CARE SETTING?

Case History

A 61-year-old woman with metastatic breast cancer is enrolled in hospice care with symptoms of ongoing pain related to metastatic bony disease for which she is receiving opioids. In recent months she has not used any laxative as her last chemotherapy regimen was associated with diarrhea. However, she is now no longer on cancer therapies and reports not having had a BM in 3 days. Which laxative(s) should this patient receive?

Suggested Answer

The management of constipation in palliative care should be individualized, keeping in mind the underlying cause(s). Opioids are frequently prescribed to palliative care patients and one of the most common cause of constipation in this patient population. While laxatives are an accepted treatment in constipation, there is no consensus on the most effective approach. In patients on opioids, a stimulant laxative such as sennoside, 1 to 2 tablets may be implemented with upward titration to 2 to 4 tablets, 2 to 3 times a day. There is now evidence to suggest that stool softeners such as docusate do not enhance the effects of sennosides alone. If constipation persists or is refractory to sennosides, osmotic agents such as lactulose or polyethylene glycol may be necessary. In the nonpalliative care population polyethylene glycol has been shown to be more effective and better tolerated than lactulose.[3] Use of suppositories and enemas should be limited to short term or when there is no systemic route. The use of mu-opioid antagonists, such as methylnaltrexone, are recommended only when traditional laxatives have not been helpful.

References

1. Tarumi Y, Wilson MP, Szafran O, Spooner GR. Randomized, double-blind, placebo-controlled trial of oral docusate in the management of constipation in hospice patients *J Pain Symptom Manage*. 2013;45:2–13.
2. Hurdon V, Viola, R., Schroder, C. How Useful is Docusate in Patients at Risk for Constipation? A Systematic Review of the Evidence in the Chronically Ill. *J Pain Symptom Manage*. 2000;19:130–136.
3. Hawley PH, Byeon JJ. A comparison of sennosides-based bowel protocols with and without docusate in hospitalized patients with cancer. *J Palliat Med*. 2008;11:575–581.
4. Candy B, Jones L, Larkin PJ, Vickerstaff V, Tookman A, Stone P. Laxatives for the management of constipation in people receiving palliative care. *Cochrane Database Syst Rev*. 2015;5:CD003448.
5. Lee-Robichaud H, Thomas K, Morgan J, Nelson RL. Lactulose versus polyethylene glycol for chronic constipation. *Cochrane Database Syst Rev*. 2010;7:CD007570.

25

Treatment of Opioid-Induced Constipation in Advanced Illness

DONNA S. ZHUKOVSKY

Subcutaneous methylnaltrexone rapidly induced laxation in patients with advanced illness and opioid-induced constipation. Treatment did not appear to affect central analgesia or precipitate opioid withdrawal.

—Thomas et al.[1]

Research Question: Is methylnaltrexone effective and safe for the treatment of opioid-induced constipation (OIC) in patients with advanced illness?

Funding: Progenics Pharmaceuticals.

Year Study Began: 2004.

Year Study Published: 2008.

Study Location: 27 US and Canadian nursing homes, hospice sites, and palliative care centers.

Who Was Studied: People 18 years of age or older with advanced illness, defined as a terminal illness such as incurable cancer or other end-stage disease; minimum life expectancy of 1 month; ≥2 week history of opioid use for analgesia; stable regimen of opioids and laxatives for ≥3 days; OIC with ≤2 bowel movements in previous week *and* no clinically meaningful laxation (investigator discretion) within 24 hours of first dose of study drug *or* no clinically meaningful laxation within 48 hours of first dose of study drug. Patients with the following were excluded: constipation not primarily caused by opioids (investigator determined), mechanical gastrointestinal obstruction, indwelling peritoneal catheter, clinically active diverticular disease, acute surgical abdomen, fecal ostomy.

How Many Patients:

- Randomized double-blind phase: 134 (106 completed)
- Open-label extension phase: 89

Study Overview: A 2-week randomized double-blind, placebo controlled trial (RCT) of study drug, followed by a 3-month open-label extension phase (Figure 25.1).

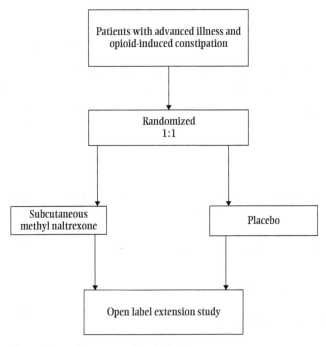

Figure 25.1 Summary of study design.

Study Intervention:

RANDOMIZED DOUBLE-BLIND PHASE
Patients were randomized to receive either subcutaneous methylnaltrexone or placebo every other day for 2 weeks. The first dose was administered by study

staff and thereafter, by a trained caregiver. Initial dosing was 0.15 mg of study drug/kilogram of body weight, with dose escalation to 0. 3mg study drug/kilogram of body weight at Day 8 if 2 or fewer rescue-free bowel movements occurred in the previous week.

Patients were allowed to continue their baseline scheduled laxative regimen and laxatives as needed, known as rescue laxatives, as long as rescue laxatives were not administered within 4 hours of the study drug.

3-MONTH OPEN-LABEL EXTENSION PHASE
Patients were allowed to continue using subcutaneous methylnaltrexone for a 3-month open-label extension phase. For this extension phase, the drug could be increased from 0.15 mg of study drug/kilogram of body weight to 0. 3mg study drug/kilogram of body weight if no bowel movement occurred within 4 hours of methylnaltrexone and decreased to 0.075 mg/kilogram of body weight if the patient experienced adverse effects after a dose of methylnaltrexone.

Follow-up: RCT (14 days); open label (3 months).

Endpoints: In the randomized phase:

Primary endpoints
1. Coprimary endpoints included the proportion of patients with rescue-free laxation within 4 hours of the first dose of the study drug as well as the proportion of patients with rescue-free laxation within 4 hours of ≥2 of the first 4 doses of the study drug.

Secondary endpoints
1. Proportion of patients with rescue-free laxation within 4 hours of ≥4 of 7 doses and within 4 hours or 24 hours after each dose
2. Proportion of patients with ≥3 laxations per week
3. Time to laxation
4. Consistency (6 categories) and difficulty (5 categories) of laxation daily
5. Overall pain scores (0–10, higher numbers more severe); current and worst in preceding 24 hours, Days 1, 7, and 14
6. Symptoms of opioid withdrawal (Modified Himmelsbach Withdrawal Scale 7–28, higher scores indicating greater severity); Days 1, 7, and 14
7. Adverse effects (National Cancer Institute's Common Toxicity Criteria version 2.0)
8. Constipation-related distress (0 = none to 4 = very much)
9. Global Clinical Impression of Change (1–7, higher scores indicating better function), Days 7 and 14 and monthly

RESULTS

- Among 134 randomized patients, 133 were included in the intention to treat analysis (62 in the methylnaltrexone group and 71 in placebo). One patient received an unblinded drug and was included only in the safety analysis.
- Participant demographics and clinical characteristics were: Median patient age (in years) for methylnaltrexone and placebo was 70 (range 38–98) and 72 (range 34–93), respectively. The total population was 57% female, 95% white, 59% primary diagnosis of cancer, 71% WHO performance status of 3 or 4.
- Baseline median (range) morphine equivalent daily dose (MEDD) was 100 (10, 160) mg for placebo versus 150 (9, 4160) mg for methylnaltrexone.
- Methylnaltrexone use was associated with a higher proportion of patients who had rescue-free laxation within 4 hours of the first dose of the study drug and within 4 hours of ≥2 doses of the first 4 doses of the study drug, as compared to placebo (48% vs. 15% and 52% vs. 8%, respectively P < 0.001 for both) (Table 25.1).

Table 25.1. EFFICACY OF METHYLNATREXONE VERSUS PLACEBO

	Methylnatrexone (n = 62)	Placebo (n = 71)	P Value
RFL within 4 hours of first dose of study drug	48%	15%	<0.0001
RFL within 4 hours of ≥2 of the first 4 doses of study drug	52%	8%	<0.0001
≥3 laxations per week	39%	6%	<0.0001
Median time to laxation	6.3 hours	>48 hours	<0.0001

NOTE: RFL = rescue-free laxation.

- Post hoc logistic regressions showed no effect of baseline MEDD, age, or performance status of cancer diagnosis on rates of rescue-free laxation.
- In responders, time to laxation was faster after methylnaltrexone than placebo. Median time to laxation after first dose 6.3 hours for methylnaltrexone versus >48 hours for placebo (Table 25.1).
- Methylnaltrexone use was associated with greater improvement in Global Clinical Impression of Change scores.
- Pain and opioid withdrawal scores showed minimal change.

- Abdominal pain, flatulence, nausea, elevated body temperature, and dizziness occurred more frequently in the methlynaltrexone group, while falls and hypotension were more common in the placebo group. None of the serious adverse events were attributed to the study drug but were considered to be related to the primary illness (Table 25.2).

Table 25.2. MOST COMMON ADVERSE EFFECTS

Adverse Event	Methylnaltrexone (n = 63)	Placebo (n = 71)
Any event	81%	80%
Abdominal pain	17%	13%
Flatulence	13%	7%
Nausea	11%	7%
Increase in body temperature	8%	3%
Dizziness	8%	3%
Pain	3%	10%
Fall	2%	10%
Hypotension	0%	6%

Criticisms and Limitations:

- Some of the evaluations of pain were conducted on study days that likely missed the time frames most at risk for pain exacerbation and accordingly may have underestimated the potentially detrimental impact of methylnaltrexone on pain intensity. Similarly, it is unclear when the evaluations of opioid withdrawal took place. Assessments for Days 1 and 7 were not timed to capture the impact of drug administration on Days 1 and 7.
- Side effects were volunteered reports and were not systematically assessed with a validated tool. While an industry standard for assessing drug-related adverse effects, this method does not capture symptoms that patients do not spontaneously volunteer and may result in underreporting. Given the gastrointestinal symptoms that commonly accompany both laxative use and constipation, a systematic evaluation of pain and gastrointestinal symptoms may have better informed drug impact on quality of life and side effects.

Other Relevant Studies and Information:

- A systematic review conducted to determine the effectiveness and differential efficacy of laxatives for management of constipation in individuals receiving palliative care found that laxatives were effective but that comparative efficacy could not be determined as the trials compared different laxatives or combinations of laxatives, precluding meta-analysis. Trials were few in number, small, and of unclear bias.[2]

- Data from a systematic review and meta-analysis of placebo-controlled trials of mu-opioid receptor antagonists (alvimopan, methylnaltrexone, naloxone, and nalbuphine) for the management of opioid-induced bowel dysfunction demonstrated improvement of gastrointestinal transit time and constipation, with side effects similar to those seen with placebo. Trials were conducted in a variety of populations and were of variable quality.[3,4] Despite improved efficacy compared to placebo, a substantial proportion of participants did not respond to the drug.
- A single-institution retrospective review of clinical usage of methylnaltrexone indicates that, outside of the trial setting, dosing errors were common and that many patients without advanced illness or those at risk for bowel perforation received the medication.[5,6] Risk-benefit ratios in these circumstances have not been established.
- The cost of methylnaltrexone is high relative to many commonly used laxatives.[7] Cost-benefit analyses to date have not yielded clear data on the cost-effectiveness of this medication.[8,9]

Summary and Implications:

- This randomized clinical trial highlights how mechanistic understanding can lead to therapeutic development, and shifts the paradigm for management of opioid-induced constipation. Methylnaltrexone is more effective than placebo for managing OIC unresponsive to initial laxative therapy among patients with advanced illness. It appears to be safe among such populations for periods of up to 4 months. Its place in the spectrum of treatments for OIC is yet to be determined and requires further study of comparative efficacy, cost-benefit analysis, and quality of life.

CLINICAL CASE: HOW TO TREAT OPIOID-INDUCED CONSTIPATION

Case History

You are asked to consult on the care of a 46-year-old woman with non-small cell lung cancer and poorly controlled pain due to chest wall involvement by tumor. She has a remote history of Hodgkin's disease and chronic constipation.

She currently uses extended and immediate relief morphine for pain but limits her use because she does not want constipation to get worse. How should you approach treating her constipation?

Suggested Answer

It would be reasonable to start by taking a history of her bowel habits prior to opioid use to establish what is "normal" for her in terms of frequency of BMs and consistency and caliber of stool, thereby providing a "target" for laxation. In addition, knowing what has been effective for her in the past and what agents have caused side effects is useful information. By establishing rapport with her and eliciting her perceptions of what has and has not worked well for her in the past, you can initiate a bowel regimen that is person-centered, and hopefully she simultaneously allows you to better titrate her opioid analgesics and employ other pharmacologic and nonpharmacologic interventions, as appropriate. For many individuals, the bowel regimen likely includes a stimulant such as senna and an agent that draws fluid into the gut, such as polyethylene glycol, to bulk up and soften the stool. However, after aggressive titration of multiple laxatives and adequate hydration, the patient still has not had a BM for 6 days and complains of nausea and bloating. At this point, the addition of methylnaltrexone or other opioid antagonists may yield improved results. From a safety perspective, it would be prudent to establish that any radiation for prior treatment of Hodgkins's disease did not include the abdomen or pelvis, that abdominal radiography shows no suspicion of bowel obstruction, and that she does not have any manifestations of intra-abdominal tumor.

References

1. Thomas J, Karver S, Cooney GA, et al. Methylnaltrexone for opioid-induced constipation in advanced illness. *N Engl J Med.* 2008;29;358:2332–2343.
2. Candy B, Jones L, Larkin PJ, Vickerstaff V, Tookman A, Stone P. Laxatives for the management of constipation in people receiving palliative care. *Cochrane Database Syst Rev.* 2015;13:CD003448.
3. McNicol ED, Boyce D, Schumann R, Carr DB. Mu-opioid antagonists for opioid-induced bowel dysfunction. *Cochrane Database Syst Rev.* 2008;16:CD006332.
4. Ford AC, Brenner DM, Schoenfeld PS. Efficacy of pharmacological therapies for the treatment of opioid-induced constipation: systematic review and meta-analysis. *Am J Gastroenterol.* 2013;108:1566–1574.
5. Watkins JL, Eckmann KR, Mace ML, Rogers J, Langley G, Smith W. Utilization of methylnaltrexone (relistor) for opioid-induced constipation in an oncology hospital. *P T.* 2011;36:33–36.
6. Mackey AC, Green L, Greene P, Avigan M. Methylnaltrexone and gastrointestinal perforation. *J Pain Symptom Manage.* 2010;40(1):e1–e3.

7. Micromedex® 1.0 (Red Book Online). Greenwood Village, CO: Truven Health Analytics. Retrieved from http://www.micromedexsolutions.com/

8. Iskedjian M, Iyer S, Librach SL, Wang M, Farah B, Berbari J. Methylnaltrexone in the treatment of opioid-induced constipation in cancer patients receiving palliative care: willingness-to-pay and cost-benefit analysis. *J Pain Symptom Manage.* 2011;41:104–115.

9. Earnshaw SR, Klok RM, Iyer S, McDade C. Methylnaltrexone bromide for the treatment of opioid-induced constipation in patients with advanced illness—a cost-effectiveness analysis. *Aliment Pharmacol Ther.* 2010;31:911–921.

26

Octreotide for Malignant Bowel Obstruction

SHALINI DALAL

> The administration of octreotide, in combination with traditional phar-
> macological treatment, can be very effective in the symptom manage-
> ment of inoperable bowel obstruction in terminal cancer patients.
> —MYSTAKIDOU ET AL.[1]

Research Question: Does octreotide help in the management of symptoms of
malignant bowel obstruction (MBO) in terminally ill patients?

Funding: Not indicated.

Year Study Began: October 1996.

Year Study Published: 2002.

Study Location: Patient homes in Athens, Greece.

Who Was Studied: Consecutive adult cancer patients with MBO who were
under the care of the Palliative Care Unit of the Areteion Hospital, Athens,
Greece.

Who Was Excluded: Patients who were deemed to benefit from surgical interventions for their MBO.

How Many Patients: 68.

Study Overview: This is a double-blinded, randomized controlled trial (RCT) in which octreotide is compared to hyoscine butylbromide for the symptomatic management of terminally ill cancer patients with MBO not amenable to surgical management (Figure 26.1).

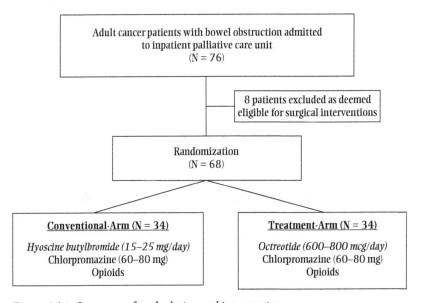

Figure 26.1 Summary of study design and intervention.

Study Intervention: Consecutive patients under the care of the palliative care team with MBO were equally randomized (34 patients each) to receive hyoscine butyl-bromide or octreotide subcutaneously (SC). Both groups received chlorpromazine SC and opioids (morphine SC or transdermal fentanyl). Nasogastric (NG) tubes and parenteral hydration were avoided. The patient's family and a member of palliative care team completed daily assessments of symptoms in a diary.

Follow-up: The research team recorded assessments at baseline, Day 3 (after start of intervention), Day 6, and a day prior to death.

Endpoints:

Primary outcomes
- Number of vomiting episodes per day
- Nausea (based on the intensity and duration of nausea in hours/day)

Secondary outcomes
- Pain intensity: 0–10 visual analogue scale by Scott-Huskisson
- Fatigue: minor or major presence
- Anorexia: minor or major presence
- Electrolyte measurements

RESULTS

- On Day 3, the octreotide arm (n = 34) as compared to the hyoscine arm (n = 34) had a higher mean percentage improvement in nausea scores from baseline (93% vs. 84%; P = 0.003).
- On Day 3, vomiting episodes was significantly better controlled in the octreotide arm as compared to the hyoscine arm (82% vs. 67.0%; P = 0.007).
- There was no statistically significant difference in nausea or vomiting symptoms between the two groups at other time points of the study (on Day 6 and 1 day before death).
- Higher improvement in fatigue from baseline scores was noted on Days 3 and 6 and prior to death for the octreotide arm as compared to the hyoscine arm.
- There was no statistically significant difference in pain and electrolytes between the two groups at any time point of the study.
- The mean doses of opioids such as morphine and fentanyl patch were lower in the octreotide arm as compared to the conventional arm.
- A higher number of patients in the hyoscine as compared to the octreotide arm dropped out of the study (12 vs. 3 patients) and required IV antiemetics, hydration, and NG tubes (NGT).
- A side effect of minor skin reaction was reported by 3 (8.8%) and 4 (11.8%) patients in the hyoscine and octreotide arm, respectively (P value not shown).

Criticisms and Limitations:

- This was a single-site study, which limits its generalizability.
- The main outcomes related to symptoms were obtained by proxy from family members and palliative care staff.
- Some important information was missing in the reporting. The paper does not describe power analysis for sample size justification, nor the procedures of randomization, blinding, or participant/proxy consent process.

Other Relevant Studies and Information:

- A recent systematic review in 2016 identified 7 RCTs that evaluated the effectiveness of somatostatin analogues (octreotide and lanreotide) compared with placebo or other agents (hyoscine butylbromide) for symptomatic relief of MBO.[2] Although a meta-analysis was not possible due to the varied design, endpoints, and timing of assessments between studies, this review concluded there was low-level evidence of benefit of somatostatin analogues (5 RCT) and high-level evidence of no benefit for symptomatic treatment of MBO (2 RCTs). In the studies reporting benefit, this benefit tended to be early during follow-up and was not sustained beyond Day 3.
- The International Conference on MBO and Clinical Protocol Committee calls for more quality research with trials using agreed-upon and clinically relevant end points.[3,4] Outcome measurements, particularly nausea and vomiting, volume of NGT secretion, along with pain and quality of life domains, need to be standardized and agreed upon to allow meaningful research in this field.

Summary and Implications: Somatostatin analogues are commonly prescribed for MBO. While some studies, including this one, demonstrated octreotide to be beneficial for the management of MBO, a recent systematic review found the data supporting a benefit for octreotide (or other somatostatins) to be equivocal and meriting further research.

CLINICAL CASE: MANAGEMENT OF BOWEL OBSTRUCTION IN PALLIATIVE CARE

Case History

A 64-year-old woman with metastatic endometrial cancer refractory to multiple treatments was recently found to have progressed on a clinical trial. She presents to the emergency center with a 3-day history of nausea, vomiting, abdominal pain, and distention. She has not had a bowel movements in 5 days. In the emergency center, the patient received IV ondansetron and morphine, which provided transient decrease in symptoms of nausea and pain, respectively. However, within an hour, the patient had another bout of emesis. Diagnostic imaging confirmed malignant small bowel obstruction, which was attributed to a progressive increase in peritoneal disease. The patient is aware that she is not a candidate for any further cancer treatment and agrees to be admitted to the palliative care unit for management of uncontrolled symptoms. How should this patient be treated?

Suggested Answer

The management of MBO should depend on the goals of treatment, location of obstruction, and overall symptoms. When appropriate, surgical interventions such as bowel resection or endoscopic stenting may be considered. However, in most terminally ill patients surgery is inappropriate and the goals of treatment should be symptom and quality of life directed. Insertion of NGT and venting G-tubes are directed toward the palliation of ongoing emesis, while medications such as octreotide *may* help with the decrease in gastrointestinal secretions and therefore allow control of future nausea and emesis. Placement of venting tubes allows patients to take small amounts of liquids and pureed diets orally, which is subsequently vented through the tubes. Management of nausea may include use of steroids or D2-antagonists such as haloperidol and chlorpromazine. Metoclopromide, a D-2 antagonist with prokinetic activity, is not recommended when MBO is complete as it may increase colicky pain but can be initiated on a trial basis in the setting of partial obstruction.

References

1. K. Mystakidou, E. Tsilika, O. Kalaidopoulou, et al. Comparison of octreotide administration vs conservative treatment in the management of inoperable bowel obstruction in patients with far advanced cancer: a randomized, double-blind, controlled clinical trial. *Anticancer Res.* 2002;22:1187–1192.
2. Obita GP, Boland EG, Currow DC, Johnson MJ, Boland JW. Somatostatin analogues compared with placebo and other pharmacologic agents in the management of symptoms of inoperable malignant bowel obstruction: a systematic review. *J Pain Symptom Manage.* 2016 Dec;52(6):901–919.
3. Anthony, T., Baron, T., Mercadante, S., et al. Report of the clinical protocol committee: development of randomized trials for malignant bowel obstruction. *J Pain Symptom Manage.* 2007;34:S49–S59.
4. Krouse, R.S. The International Conference on Malignant Bowel Obstruction: a meeting of the minds to advance palliative care research. *J Pain Symptom Manage.* 2007;34:S1–S6.

Psychosocial Aspects of
Care and Communication

27

Prevalence of Mood Disorders in Patients with Cancer

LINH NGUYEN

Interview-defined depression and anxiety is less common in patients with cancer than previously thought, although some combination of mood disorders occurs in 30–40% of patients in hospital settings without a significant difference between palliative care and non-palliative care settings.

—MITCHELL ET AL.[1]

Research Question: (1) In oncological, haematological and palliative care settings, what is the prevalence of depression, anxiety, and adjustment disorders based on diagnostic interviews? (2) In these settings, what are the predictors of the presence of depression?

Funding: None.

Year Study Published: 2011.

Study Location: Not applicable.

Who Was Studied: This meta-analysis included studies involving a mental health assessment by psychiatric interview of adults with cancer in hospital settings.

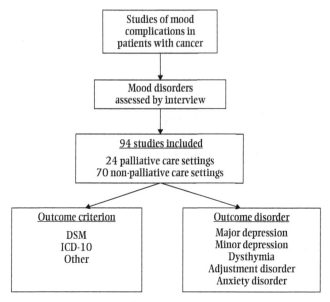

Figure 27.1 Summary of study selection.

Who Was Excluded: Studies using epidemiologically selective samples (e.g., intervention trials), those with study participants under the age of 18, studies with prevalence of depression in patients before the diagnosis of cancer, duplicate publications (i.e., studies investigating the same sample), community surveys because the authors considered the sample to be too small and clinically distinct, and studies with no primary data and insufficient data for analysis were excluded.

How Many Patients: 433 studies of mood disorders in patients with cancer.

Study Overview: Using the Preferred Reporting Items for Systematic Reviews and Meta-Analyses (PRISMA) guidelines, the first and last authors designed the protocol and extraction forms. They performed a systematic search of abstract databases including Medline, PsycINFO, and Embase from beginning to 2010. They searched four full-text collections and contacted authors of publications for primary data when necessary (Figure 27.1).

Three authors independently extracted the data and assigned a 4-point quality rating and a 5-point bias risk to each study. The quality rating considered the sample size, study design, attrition rate, criterion method, and the dealing with possible confounders. The bias rating considered possible biases in age, gender, clinical setting, and cancer type and stage. Each study's sampling method was evaluated because it could affect the interpretation of prevalence. The first and last authors resolved differences.

Study Intervention: Not applicable.

Follow-up: Not applicable.

Endpoints: Main outcome: syndromal (clinical) depression defined by formal interview and using *Diagnostic and Statistical Manual of Mental Disorders* (DSM) research criteria for major depression, minor depression, dysthymia, adjustment disorder (either alone or in combination with depression), anxiety disorders, and combined mood disorders. Secondary outcome: correlates of depression.

RESULTS

- The investigators identified 369 articles that included patients with cancer who were assessed by interview-based diagnostic methods (Table 27.1).

Table 27.1. SUMMARY OF STUDY'S KEY FINDINGS

	Palliative Care Settings	Oncological and Haematological Settings
Studies	24	70
Patients	4,007	10,071
Countries	7	14
Prevalence		
All types of depression combined	24.6%	20.7%
Depression or adjustment disorder	24.7%	31.6%
All types of mood disorders	29%	38.2%
Unitary Diagnoses		
DSM- or ICD-defined depression	16.5%	16.3%
DSM-defined major depression	14.3%	14.9%
DSM-defined minor depression	9.6%	19.2%
Adjustment disorder	15.4%	19.4%
Anxiety disorder	9.8%	10.3%
Dysthymia	Insufficient sample	2.7%

NOTE: DSM = *Diagnostic and Statistical Manual of Mental Disorders*; ICD = International Classification of Diseases.

- In both palliative care settings and oncological and haematological settings, there was no association between age and gender and the prevalence of depression or anxiety. However, in the palliative care settings, there was a small association between women and adjustment disorder (adjusted r^2 0.06, P = 0.02).
- In the oncological and haematological settings, high study quality was associated with low prevalence of depression (P = 0.003).

Criticisms and Limitations:

- When compared to self-report scales, interviews commonly underestimate the prevalence of psychiatric disorders.
- Because of the paucity of long-term data, the authors noted that their results might only represent the first 5 years after diagnosis. The authors noted that they would have liked to examine the effect of the stage of treatment and disease duration on the prevalence of depression.
- Correlates of depression and anxiety could not be extracted due to the data set. Other predictors of depression and adjustment disorder such as low performance status, high symptom burden, previous depression, and low levels of support were not examined.

Other Relevant Studies and Information:

- Other studies have reported the prevalence of depression as ranging from 0% to 38% in patients with cancer and 5% to 26% in patients in palliative care settings.[2,3] Differences between these rates and those reported here may result from differences in study population, criteria used to define depression, and rigor of the assessment.
- A 12-month study examining the prevalence of major depression in the hospital setting among patients in the community reported similar results as this one.[4]
- In cancer patients with moderate to severe depression at least half are willing to accept professional help or referral.[5,6]

Summary and Implications: This study found that approximately 21% to 25% of patients with cancer suffer from mood disorders. Given the high prevalence, it is important for clinicians to screen for these conditions and to be familiar with the appropriate management. In addition to depression, clinicians should remain attentive to related mood complications including adjustment and anxiety disorders.

CLINICAL CASE: DOES THIS PATIENT HAVE MAJOR DEPRESSIVE DISORDER?

Case History

An 85-year-old man with advanced prostate cancer reports depressed mood and lack of joy for 2 months and feeling hopeless, and he wants to end his life. The patient also reports a decrease in appetite, difficulty in falling asleep, feeling fatigued, and low energy. The patient also has significant pain due to bony metastases.

What is the most likely diagnosis, and which symptoms support the diagnosis?

Suggested Answer

The most likely diagnosis is major depressive disorder, single episode. Five of nine symptoms for more than 2 weeks are required to make the diagnosis, and depressed mood or anhedonia must be one of the symptoms. The somatic signs and symptoms of DSM-defined major depressive disorder are less valuable because the cancer itself can produce fatigue, diminished energy, anorexia, and insomnia.

The differential diagnosis of depressed mood includes normal grief and untreated pain. However, thoughts of hastened death point to a diagnosis of major depressive disorder. Differentiating major depression from normal grief and expected emotional distress is challenging, and patients who do not meet the diagnostic criteria for major depressive disorder will not likely benefit from pharmacological interventions.

References

1. Mitchell AJ, Chan M, Bhatti H, et al. Prevalence of depression, anxiety, and adjustment disorder in oncological, haematological, and palliative-care settings: a meta-analysis of 94 interview-based studies. *Lancet Oncol.* 2011;12(2):160–174. doi:10.1016/S1470-2045(11)70002-X

2. Massie MJ. Prevalence of depression in patients with cancer. *JNCI Monographs.* 2004;2004(32):57–71. doi:10.1093/jncimonographs/lgh014

3. Hotopf M, Chidgey J, Addington-Hall J, Ly KL. Depression in advanced disease: a systematic review, part 1: prevalence and case finding. *Palliat Med.* 2002;16(2):81–97.

4. Rasic DT, Belik S, Bolton JM, Chochinov HM, Sareen J. Cancer, mental disorders, suicidal ideation and attempts in a large community sample. *Psychooncology.* 2008;17(7):660–667. doi:10.1002/pon.1292

5. Endicott J. Measurement of depression in patients with cancer. *Cancer.* 1984;53(10 Suppl.):2243–2249.
6. Curry C, Cossich T, Matthews JP, Beresford J, McLachlan SA. Uptake of psychosocial referrals in an outpatient cancer setting: improving service accessibility via the referral process. *Supportive Care Cancer.* 2002;10(7):549–555. doi:10.1007/s00520-002-0371-2

28

Dignity Therapy for Patients Near the End of Life

MARVIN OMAR DELGADO-GUAY

Dignity therapy is a feasible and effective intervention to address suffering in patients toward the end-of-life.

—CHOCHINOV ET AL.[1]

Research Question: Is it feasible and effective to provide an individualized psychotherapeutic intervention, dignity therapy, to address psychosocial and existential distress among terminally ill patients?

Funding: Cancer Council of Western Australia, American Foundation for Suicide Prevention, National Cancer Institute of Canada, Canadian Cancer Society, and the Canadian Institutes for Health Research.

Year Study Began: 2001.

Year Study Published: 2005.

Study Location: Silver Chain Hospice Care Service (Osborne Park, Western Australia, Australia), the Cancer Council Centre for Palliative Care Cottage Hospice (Shenton Park, Western Australia, Australia), and Winnipeg Regional Health Authority Palliative Care Program (Winnipeg, Manitoba, Canada).

Who Was Studied: Patients with (1) terminal illness associated with a life expectancy of less than 6 months; (2) minimum age of 18 years; (3) English speaking; (4) a commitment to three to four contacts over approximately 7 to 10 days; and (5) willingness to provide verbal and written consent.

Who Was Excluded: Those with cognitive impairment based on clinical consensus.

How Many Patients: 100.

Study Overview: This is a prospective single-arm phase II trial with a before/after comparison. Eligible patients with terminal illness were asked to complete a series of psychometric assessments evaluating physical, psychological, and existential outcomes before the intervention was delivered. All patients received the dignity therapy intervention (see later description). After the session, patients completed the same psychometric assessments (Figure 28.1). Analysis was performed comparing assessments pre- and post-dignity therapy.

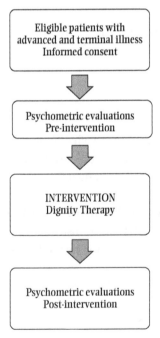

Figure 28.1 Summary of study design.

Study Intervention: Dignity Therapy is a psychotherapy based in the model of Dignity in Palliative Care that involves generativity, continuity of self, preservation of self, maintenance of pride, hopefulness, aftermath concerns, and care tenor. The patients were first interviewed based on a manualized protocol by a psychiatrist, psychologist, or palliative care nurse. Typically, one session was conducted over 30 to 60 minutes, although up to 3 sessions were sometimes required. The therapy sessions were taped, transcribed verbatim, and edited, and the dialogue was then transformed to a narrative over 2 to 3 days. The edited transcript was then immediately returned and read to the patients, who were given the opportunity to make further editing or additions if needed. The entire process was typically completed within 10 days.

Follow-up: Not applicable.

Endpoints:
- Feasibility of dignity therapy (primary endpoint): Single-item 7-point ordinal scales to examine sense of dignity, depression, anxiety, suffering, hopefulness, desire for death, suicidality, and sense of well-being. This screening approaches yield interrater (0.92–0.97) and test–retest (0.50–0.90) reliability[2] and correlated highly with their visual analog equivalent (0.78 to 90).[3] Also, it used a 2-item quality of life instrument.[4]
- Revised Edmonton Symptom Assessment Scale with 10 items that ranged from 0 to 10, with an addition of will-to live visual analog scale.[5]
- Postintervention dignity therapy satisfaction survey

RESULTS

- 100 patients completed the study in both sites: 50 patients from Australia and 50 from Canada.
- The mean age of patients was 63.9 years (range 22–95; standard deviation 14.2), and 44 were women; 97% of the patients had cancer. The patients' religious affiliations were Protestant (34%), Catholic (23%), Jewish (2%), other (16%), and no religious affiliation (24%).
- The median length of survival from the time of the initial interview to the time of death was 51 days (range 3–377). The median survival from the time that the generativity document was received to the time of death was 40 days (range 0–371).
- Qualitative analyses showed that 91% of participants reported that they were satisfied or highly satisfied with the intervention; 86% reported that the intervention was helpful or very helpful.

- There were improvement in patients' sense of dignity (67%), increased sense of purpose (68%), increased sense of meaning (67%), and increased will to live (47%). Eighty-one percent of patients believed that dignity therapy helped or would have helped their family members.
- There was improvement in dignity postintervention. There was significant improvement of measures of suffering in self-reports of depressed mood (Table 28.1).

Table 28.1. IMPROVEMENT IN MEASURES
POST–DIGNITY THERAPY

Measures	One-Tailed P Value
Suffering	0.023
Depressed mood	0.05
Dignity	0.085

- Hopelessness, desire for death, anxiety, will to live, and suicide all showed nonsignificant changes favoring improvement.
- Patients who found dignity therapy helpful correlated with feeling that it had made life currently feel more meaningful ($r = 0.566$; $P < 0.0001$), heightening sense of purpose ($r = 0.547$; $P < 0.0001$), decreasing suffering ($r = 0.267$; $P < 0.008$), and increasing will to live ($r = 0.290$; $P < 0.004$).
- Patients who believed that dignity therapy had helped or would be of help to their family correlated significantly with life feeling more meaningful ($r = 0.480$; $P < 0.0001$) and having a sense of purpose ($r = 0.562$; $P < 0.0001$) and was accompanied by a decreased sense of suffering ($r = 0.327$; $P < 0.001$) and increased will to live ($r = 0.387$; $P < 0.0001$).

Criticisms and Limitations:

- This trial was conducted as a single-arm feasible study in which all the patients received the intervention without comparison against standard of care or other intervention. Without a control group, it is unclear how much placebo effect could have affected the patient-reported outcomes.
- The definition for feasibility was not clearly outlined. Among 129 patients enrolled, however, the completion rate was 78%, and a majority found the intervention to be helpful.
- Other than the revised Edmonton Symptom Assessment Scale, the measures to assess many secondary outcomes such as suffering, hopefulness, desire of death, suicide, and sense of well-being have not been validated. There was also limited reporting of the values of these

outcomes in the manuscript, making it challenging to understand the magnitude of change.

Other Information and Relevant Studies:

- The three major categories were dignity-conserving repertoire, illness-related concerns, and social dignity inventory.[6]
- In a study of 213 palliative care patients, Chochinov et al. found that 16 (7.5%) indicated that loss of dignity was a great concern. These patients were more likely to experience psychological and symptom distress, had heightened dependency needs, and showed loss of will to live.[7]
- A recent systematic review involving 5 randomized trials concluded that there was some evidence to support that dignity therapy could improve anxiety and depression, particularly among patients with a high baseline level of psychological distress.[8]
- A survey of 60 family members of patients who took part in this study found that they perceived the dignity therapy generativity document to be helpful for the patient and for themselves.[9]

Summary and Implications:

- This study suggests that dignity therapy is feasible among dying patients and may be associated with favorable outcomes. Dignity therapy is now being implemented in an increasing number of centers worldwide.

CLINICAL CASE: HOW CAN WE HELP PATIENTS WITH LIFE-THREATENING ILLNESS WITH EXISTENTIAL SUFFERING? WHO CAN BENEFIT FROM DIGNITY THERAPY?

Case History

Mr. JR is a patient with advanced and progressive carcinoma. He had received several lines of treatment, but unfortunately his illness has continued to progress. This has caused him a debilitated and frail life. He used to be a well-known worker, respected by his colleagues, and loved by his family. While he has developed several physical distressful symptoms, he also has a sense of loneliness and feeling that his enjoyment in life has vanished. Even though he knows that his family cares for and loves him, he does not want to be a burden to them; he has preferred not to share what he has been going through with this illness and how much control in his life has disappeared. Even his relationship with the higher power has changed, and he is questioning his own existence, although not expressing suicidal ideations. Our role in caring for this patient is to control his physical, emotional, and spiritual suffering. Providing expressive supportive counseling might help him as well. Can we use other psychotherapeutic intervention, considering his frail status, that can help him to boost his distressful life?

Suggested Answer

Dignity therapy is a feasible and potentially effective intervention to address suffering in patients toward the end of life,[1] and it would be advisable to provide dignity therapy to this patient.

Living with an illness that affects our integrity and dignity as human beings and facing our own mortality can lead us to develop a spiritual/existential crisis.[2,3] One of the greatest challenges facing palliative medicine today is how to attend to those patients whose anguish resides beyond the scope of conventional symptom distress.[4,5] For many palliative care patients, their families, and their caregivers, "dignity" conveys an inherent respect to be granted patients in preparation for death.[6-8]

The ultimate goal of dignity therapy is to help bolster the dignity of dying patients and mitigate the effects of their suffering. The basic components involving the dignity therapy include generativity/legacy, maintaining hope, continuity of self, maintenance of pride and role preservation, autonomy/control, living the moment, social support, aftermath concerns, and care tenor.

References

1. Chochinov HM, Hack T, Hassard T, Kristjanson LJ, McClement S, Harlos M. Dignity therapy: a novel psychotherapeutic intervention for patients near the end of life. *J Clin Oncol*. 2005 Aug 20;23(24):5520–5525.
2. Wilson KG, Grahan ID, Viola RA, et al. Structured interview assessment of symptoms and concerns in palliative care. *Can J Psychiatry*. 2004;49:350–358.
3. Breitbart W, Rosenfeld BD, Passik SD. Interest in physician-assisted suicide among ambulatory HIV-infected patients. *Am J Psychiatry*. 1996;153:238–242.
4. Graham KY, Longman AJ. Quality of life in persons with melanoma: preliminary model testing. *Cancer Nurs*. 1987;10:338–346.
5. Bruera E, Kuehn N, Miller MJ, et al. The Edmonton Symptom Assessment System (ESAS): a simple method for the assessment of palliative care patients. *J Palliat Care*. 1991;7:6–9.
6. Chochinov HM, Hack T, McClement S, et al. Dignity in the terminally ill: an empirical model. *Soc Sci Med*. 2002;54:433–443.

7. Chochinov HM, Hack T, Hassard T, et al. Dignity in the terminally ill: a cross-sectional cohort study. *Lancet*. 2002;360:2026–2030.
8. Martínez M, Arantzamendi M, Belar A, et al. "Dignity therapy," a promising intervention in palliative care: a comprehensive systematic literature review. *Palliat Med*. 2017;31(6):492–509.
9. McClement S, Chochinov HM, Hack T, Hassard T, Kristjanson LJ, Harlos M. Dignity therapy: family member perspectives. *J Palliat Med*. 2007;10(5):1076–1082.

29

Association between Spirituality/Religiosity and Quality of End-of-Life Care

MARVIN OMAR DELGADO-GUAY

> Religious coping in advanced cancer patients is associated with receipt of intensive life-prolonging medical care near death.
>
> —PHELPS ET AL.[1]

Research Question: How does religious coping relate to the use of intensive life-prolonging end-of-life care among patients with advanced cancer?

Funding: National Cancer Institute and National Institute of Mental Health.

Year Study Began: 2003.

Year Study Published: 2009.

Study Location: Yale Cancer Center (New Haven, CT), Veterans' Affairs Connecticut Healthcare System Comprehensive Cancer Clinics (West Haven, CT), Simmons Comprehensive Cancer Care Center (Dallas, TX), Parkland Hospital Palliative Care Service (Dallas, TX), Massachusetts General Hospital (Boston, MA), Dana-Farber Cancer Institute (Boston, MA), and New Hampshire Oncology-Hematology (Hookset, NH).

Who Was Studied: Patients with (1) a diagnosis of an advanced cancer with metastases; (2) disease progression following first-line chemotherapy; (3) age at least 20 years; (4) presence of an informal caregiver (e.g., spouse); (5) adequate stamina to complete the 45-minute interview; and (6) ability to speak either English or Spanish.

Who Was Excluded: Patients with cognitive impairment determined by neurobehavioral cognitive status examination.

How Many Patients: 345.

Study Overview: This was a prospective longitudinal cohort study. Patients completed various assessments at baseline, including the Brief RCOPE questionnaire that assesses spiritual coping, Brief COPE questionnaire, McGill Quality of Life Questionnaire, care preferences (comfort vs. long prolongation), and advance care planning (do-not-resuscitate orders, living will, health care proxy/durable power of attorney). Using the Brief RCOPE, a high positive religious coping was defined as a score at or above the median (i.e., 12 out of 21 points) (Figure 29.1).

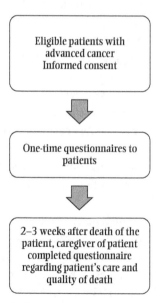

Figure 29.1 Summary of study design.

Study Intervention: None.

Follow-up: Patients were followed until death, a median of 122 days after baseline assessment. Within 2 to 3 weeks after death, caregivers most involved in the patients' care were contacted to provide information on end-of-life care and quality of death.

Endpoints: The primary outcome was intensive life-prolonging care, defined as receipt of ventilation or resuscitation during the last week of life. Secondary outcomes were hospice enrolment and death in the intensive care unit (ICU).

RESULTS

- The study sample was restricted to 345 deceased participants with postmortem data and complete baseline assessments of coping.
- Among these included patients, 79% reported that religion helped them to cope to a moderate extent or more; 32% reported that it was the most important thing that kept them going; and 56% engaged in prayer/meditation/religious study at least daily.
- 52% of participants had high positive religious coping based on study definition. Higher levels of positive religious coping was significantly associated with being black or Hispanic ($p < 0.001$), younger, less education, less likely to be insured, less likely to be married, and more likely to be recruited from Texas.
- High positive religious coping was associated with preference for heroic measures (38% vs. 9%, odds ratio [OR] = 6.6, P < 0.001) and lower likelihood of having a living will (29% vs. 68%, OR = 0.2, P < 0.001), medical power of attorney (34% vs. 64%, OR = 0.29, P < 0.001), and do-not resuscitate order (34% vs. 49%, OR = 0.53, P = 0.004).
- Higher level of positive religious coping was associated with more intensive care in the last week of life and greater likelihood of death in the ICU (Table 29.1).
- The relationship between high positive religious coping and intensive life-prolonging care remained significant after controlling for other coping methods (adjusted OR [AOR] = 3.2; 95% confidence interval [CI] 1.24–8.30), terminal illness acknowledgement, and support of spiritual needs (AOR = 2.94; 95% CI 1.13–7.63), and preference for heroics and completion of advance directives (AOR = 2.65; 95% CI 1.00–7.00).

Table 29.1. Religious Coping and End-of-Life Care

End-of-Life Care Preferences	High Religious Coping (%)	Low Religious Coping (%)	Adjusted OR (95% Confidence Interval)
Intensive life-prolonging care	13.6	4.2	2.90 (1.14–7.35)
Mechanical ventilation	11.3	3.6	2.81 (1.03–7.69)
Resuscitation	7.4	1.8	3.05 (0.79–11.78)
Death in ICU	10.7	4.2	1.80 (0.68–4.73)
Hospice care enrollment	71.3	73.5	0.97 (0.58–1.65)

NOTE: OR = odds ratio; ICU = intensive care unit.

Criticisms and Limitations:

- This was a multicenter study from different geographical locations in United States and ~70% of the patients were Christians. Thus the study findings may not be generalizable to other countries or other religions.
- The median was used to define high versus low positive religious coping; however, religious coping occurs on a spectrum.
- This was a one-time survey; however, religious coping may vary in intensity over the course of illness.

Other Relevant Studies and Information:

- The Coping with Cancer Study found that 88% of patients felt that religion was very important or somewhat important. Patients in this study also reported that 47% and 72% of the religious communities and medical communities, respectively, supported their spiritual needs to a small extent or not at all.[2]
- In another report from the Coping with Cancer Study, negative religious coping was associated with suicidal ideation (AOR 2.65, 95% CI 1.22–5.74).[3]
- Another analysis from the Coping with Cancer study found that a greater degree of spiritual care provided by the medical team was associated with greater hospice use at the end of life (AOR = 4.93, 95% CI 1.64–14.80) and less aggressive care at the end of life (AOR = 0.18, 95% CI 0.04–0.79) among high religious coping patients but not patients with low religious coping.[4]

• Furthermore, the Coping with Cancer Study found that community spiritual care was associated with more aggressive care at the end of life (AOR 5.22, 95% CI 1.71–15.60) and less likely to enroll in hospice (AOR 0.37, 95% CI 0.20–0.70).[5]

Summary and Implications: This well-designed study provides convincing evidence on how religiosity and spiritual care can impact patient preferences, decision-making, and, ultimately, end-of-life care outcomes. Specifically, a high rate of religiosity seems to be related to increased rates of receipt of aggressive end-of-life care.

CLINICAL CASE: RECOGNIZING THE IMPORTANCE OF SPIRITUALITY AND RELIGIOSITY AND COPING STRATEGIES AND END-OF-LIFE MEDICAL DECISIONS

Case History

Mr. OR is a 53-year-old man with progressive and debilitated life-threatening illness. He has poor performance status. When discussing that he is not a candidate for further treatment for his illness, he begins to cry. His wife is also tearful. He has expressed strong faith in God and tells you that he is not ready to give up. He believes that God is going to cure him and many people in his church are praying for him. Only God will decide when to stop. How do you proceed?

Suggested Answer

Spiritual and religious beliefs can affect the way patients cope with illness-related stress and disease burden. Suffering is a biopsychosocial, multidimensional construct that includes physical, emotional, and spiritual pain/struggles.[3] When spiritual needs and spiritual distress are not addressed, patients are at risk of depression and reduced sense of spiritual meaning, peace, and dignity, and the caregiver also suffers.[4-6] Facing a life-threatening illness and the end-of-life can be a spiritual crisis.

As shown in the Coping with Cancer Study, religious coping may be associated with desire for more aggressive interventions at the end of life and adverse clinical outcomes. At the same time, appropriate spiritual care from the medical team may attenuate this effect.

After acknowledging and validating his emotions, worries, and fears, the medical team including the chaplain continues to talk with the patient about his relationship with God and what God has given him in his life, allowing him to identify the most important thing that he wants to accomplish at this moment in his life. As he is able to express and share with the team his wishes, the patient also expresses acceptance and feels at peace with his condition and the proximity of death. Later the patient accepts hospice and feels at peace surrounded by his family and friends.

References

1. Phelps AC, Maciejewski PK, Nilson M, et al. Association between religious coping and use of intensive life prolonging care near death among patients with advanced cancer. *JAMA*. 2009 March 18;301(11):1140–1147.
2. Balboni TA, Vanderwerker LC, Block SD, et al. Religiousness and spiritual support among advanced cancer patients and associations with end-of-life treatment preferences and quality of life. *J Clin Oncol*. 2007;25(5):555–560.
3. Trevino KM1, Balboni M, Zollfrank A, Balboni T, Prigerson HG. Negative religious coping as a correlate of suicidal ideation in patients with advanced cancer. *Psychooncology*. 2014 Aug;23(8):936–945.
4. Balboni TA, Paulk ME, Balboni MJ, et al. Provision of spiritual care to patients with advanced cancer: associations with medical care and quality of life near death. *J Clin Oncol*. 2010;28(3):445–452.
5. Balboni TA, Balboni M, Enzinger AC, et al. Provision of spiritual support to patients with advanced cancer by religious communities and associations with medical care at the end-of-life. *JAMA Intern Med*. 2013 Jun 24;173(12):1109–1117.

The Study to Understand Prognoses and Preferences for Outcomes and Risks of Treatments (SUPPORT)

NATHAN A. GRAY AND THOMAS W. LEBLANC

> [This study] confirmed substantial shortcomings in care for seriously ill hospitalized adults.
>
> —SUPPORT PRINCIPAL INVESTIGATORS[1]

Research Question: Can timely and reliable prognostic information as well as structured avenues for communication about end-of-life preferences reduce the frequency of a painful, mechanically supported, or prolonged process of dying?

Funding: Robert Wood Johnson Foundation.

Year Study Began: 1989.

Year Study Published: 1995.

Study Location: 5 academic medical centers.

Who Was Studied: Inpatients with advanced stages of one of nine illnesses (acute respiratory failure, multiple organ system failure from sepsis, multiple organ system failure from malignancy, coma, chronic obstructive lung disease, congestive heart failure, cirrhosis, metastatic colon cancer, and non-small cell lung cancer).

Who Was Excluded: Patients who were younger than 18 years old, admitted to the psychiatric ward, died within 48 hours after hospital admission, scheduled to discharge in <72 hours, did not speak English, had AIDS, were pregnant, or had suffered a burn or trauma.

How Many Patients: Phase I: 4,301; Phase II: 4,804.

Study Overview: See Figure 30.1 for a summary of the study design.

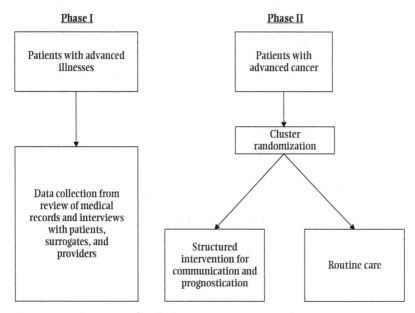

Figure 30.1 Summary of study design.

1. Phase I was a prospective observational study aimed at collecting information regarding the process of decision-making and patient outcomes. Data were collected from both concurrent and retrospective review of medical records and interviews with patients, surrogates, and physicians. The objective of phase I was to identify barriers to optimal management and shortcomings in patient–physician communication for seriously ill hospitalized adults and to develop the predictive models for use in phase II.

2. Phase II was a cluster-randomized, controlled clinical trial in which 4,804 patients were randomized (based on the specialty of their attending physician) to either a structured intervention for prognostication and communication or to control (standard care). Randomizing by physician rather than patient reduced the risk of contamination that otherwise might occur if a particular physician had patients in both the intervention and control groups.

Study Intervention: The physicians of patients in the intervention group were provided estimates of 6-month survival, outcomes of cardiopulmonary resuscitation, and functional disability at 6 months, based on the SUPPORT prognostic model.[2] (This model was based on diagnosis, number of days in the hospital, presence of cancer, neurologic function, and 11 physiologic measures.) They also received reports of the symptoms and preferences of the patient and family from interviews. In most cases, the information that the study generated was placed openly in the medical record. A trained nurse then engaged in multiple contacts with the family, patient, physician, and hospital staff to elicit patient preferences, improve understanding of outcomes, promote pain control, and facilitate advance care planning and patient-doctor communication.

Follow-up: At 6 months and following patient's death.

Endpoints: (1) Incidence and timing of do-not-resuscitate (DNR) orders; (2) patient and physician agreement on preference to withhold resuscitation; (3) days spent in an intensive care unit (ICU), receiving mechanical ventilation, or comatose before death; (4) frequency of and severity of pain; (5) hospital resource utilization.

RESULTS

- Phase I: Less than half (47%) of physicians knew when their patients wished not to have cardiopulmonary resuscitation (CPR); 38% of patients spent at least 10 days in an ICU; and for 50% of patients who died in the hospital, family members reported moderate to severe pain at least half of the time. Nearly half (46%) of DNR orders were written within 2 days of death (Table 30.1).
- Phase II: Despite the study intervention, patients experienced no improvement in patient–physician communication, nor in the five primary outcome measures described earlier. The intervention did not reduce the use of hospital resources.

Table 30.1. SUMMARY OF STUDY'S KEY FINDINGS—EFFECT OF PHASE II
INTERVENTION ON TARGET ENDPOINTS

	Adjusted Ratio (Intervention vs. Control Group)	95% CI
Time until DNR was written (median days)	1.02	0.90–1.15
DNR agreement between physicians and patients (percentage)	1.22	0.99–1.49
Time spent in undesirable states (ICU, mechanical ventilation, coma; median days)	0.97	0.87–1.07
Pain (percentage)	1.15	1.00–1.33
Resource Use (median dollars)	1.05	0.99–1.12

NOTE: CI = confidence interval; DNR = do not resuscitate; ICU = intensive care unit.

Criticisms and Limitations:

- The trial was broad in scope but designed to test improvements in decision-making rather than end-of-life care per se.
- Physicians did not receive specific training in pain management, and no standardized pain treatment protocol was provided. Thus, even if they were aware that their patients were in pain, they may not have offered effective interventions.
- Multiple explanations for the study's negative findings have been proposed, including its use of a study nurse (without required attending physician involvement), variability in the degree of intervention from communication facilitators, and limitation of the intervention to involvement only in the hospital setting.[3]
- Ultimately, the study focused on a communication intervention alone; the ineffectiveness of such a rigorously designed intervention points to the inherent complexity in decision-making as well as to the influence of broader environmental and cultural factors on practices at the end of life.[4]

Other Relevant Studies and Information:

- The context has changed substantially since SUPPORT was done. Only one of the SUPPORT hospitals had a palliative care consult program, and decisions against potentially beneficial treatments (and even hospice) were still novel at the time of the study. This study contributed valuable baseline data for the future study of care at the end of life.

- A subsequent randomized trial of communication facilitators in ICU patients with >30% predicted mortality was found to decrease ICU costs and length of stay among decedents. The intervention also improved family depressive symptoms, although it did not improve anxiety or posttraumatic stress disorder (PTSD).[5]
- Conversely, another recent trial of routine family informational and emotional support meetings (conducted by an outside facilitator) for patients with prolonged mechanical ventilation did not reduce family anxiety or depressive symptoms and may have increased PTSD symptoms. The intervention did not influence hospital length of stay.[6]
- While results of studies using communication facilitators have been mixed, a randomized trial of the effect of palliative care teams showed cost reduction, fewer ICU stays, and greater patient satisfaction.[7] Additionally, a systematic review of multiple intervention types concluded that consultation from ethics or palliative care teams or structured communication from the primary team could reduce ICU length of stay and intensity of care and improve family emotional outcomes.[8]

Summary and Implications: Communication at the end of life is extremely complex, and many patients experience prolonged care under circumstances that may conflict with their preferences. While detailed prognostic information and facilitated communication in this trial did not impact end-of-life outcomes, this study provided extensive descriptive baseline data and established the foundation for future end-of-life research by demonstrating that studies of this scale and complexity were feasible.

CLINICAL CASE: HOW SHOULD A HOSPITAL ADMINISTRATOR ALLOCATE FUNDING?

Case History
A suburban hospital in St. Paul, Minnesota, is looking for ways to improve outcomes for patients admitted with advanced illness and has just received a large donation from a local philanthropist. One administrator suggests devoting the funds to a new program that will facilitate communication by hiring a coordinator to provide structured meetings and prognostic information in the ICU. Would this be money well spent?

Suggested Answer

While an intervention offering a facilitator for routine, structured prognostication and communication would intuitively seem to promote matching care to patient preferences and reduce the utilization of costly or painful treatments at the end of life, interventions focused only on communication support via an external facilitator have not consistently delivered such improvements. This phenomenon could be attributable to numerous variables, including lack of continuity or an absence of trust when outside facilitators lead communication and the lack of trained professionals to deliver effective interventions.

Nonetheless, mounting evidence suggests that the communication and interdisciplinary support provided by palliative care teams does have a meaningful impact on patient outcomes and health utilization, compared to more limited communication interventions. Future study may clarify the primary means by which such teams impact care or may better match patients to the types of communication support that will be most useful; presently, this hospital might be better served using the funds toward implementation of a full palliative care team rather than an isolated communication intervention.

References

1. SUPPORT Principal Investigators. A controlled trial to improve care for seriously ill hospitalized patients: the study to understand prognoses and preferences for outcomes and risks of treatments (SUPPORT). *JAMA.* 1995;274(20):1591–1598.

2. Knaus WA, Harrell FE Jr., Lynn J, et al. The SUPPORT prognostic model: objective estimates of survival for seriously ill hospitalized adults. Study to Understand Prognoses and Preferences for Outcomes and Risks of Treatments. *Ann Intern Med.* 1995;122(3):191–203.

3. Lynn J, De Vries KO, Arkes HR, et al. Ineffectiveness of the SUPPORT intervention: review of explanations. *J Am Geriatr Soc* 2000;48(5 Suppl.):S206–S213.

4. Lynn J, Arkes HR, Stevens M, et al. Rethinking fundamental assumptions: SUPPORT's implications for future reform. Study to Understand Prognoses and Preferences and Risks of Treatment. *J Am Geriatr Soc* 2000; 48(5 Suppl):S214–S221.

5. Curtis JR, Treece PD, Nielsen EL, et al. Randomized trial of communication facilitators to reduce family distress and intensity of end-of-life care. *Am J Respir Crit Care Med.* 2015;193(2):154–162.

6. Carson SS, Cox CE, Wallenstein S, et al. Effect of palliative care–led meetings for families of patients with chronic critical illness: a randomized clinical trial. *JAMA.* 2016;316(1):51–62.

7. Gade G, Venohr I, Conner D, et al. Impact of an inpatient palliative care team: a randomized control trial. *J Palliat Med.* 2008;11(2):180–190.

8. Scheunemann LP, McDevitt M, Carson SS, Hanson LC. Randomized, controlled trials of interventions to improve communication in intensive care: a systematic review. *Chest.* 2011;139(3):543–554.

31

Doctors' Prognostic Accuracy
in Terminally Ill Patients

ANJALI DESAI AND ANDREW S. EPSTEIN

> Doctors are inaccurate in their prognoses for terminally ill patients and
> the error is systematically optimistic.
>
> —CHRISTAKIS AND LAMONT[1]

Research Question: Are doctors' prognoses accurate in terminally ill patients,
and what factors are associated with prognostic accuracy?

Funding: Soros Foundation Project on Death in America Faculty Scholars
Program, the American Medical Association Education and Research
Foundation, Robert Wood Johnson Clinical Scholars Program.

Year Study Began: 1996.

Year Study Published: 2000.

Study Location: 5 outpatient hospice programs in Chicago, IL.

Who Was Studied: Patients admitted to these hospice programs during 130
consecutive days in 1996, as well as their referring physicians.

Who Was Excluded: Children, patients and physicians who refused to give consent, patients who died before study investigators were notified about the patient or before the referring physician could be contacted, patients who had missing dates of death by the study's conclusion, referring physicians who could not be contacted.

How Many Patients: 468 patients and 343 referring physicians.

Study Overview: This is a prospective cohort study. Physicians were asked to provide an estimate of patient survival at the time of hospice referral. The accuracy of prognostication was assessed by comparing the estimated survival against actual survival. Patient and physician characteristics associated with accuracy of prognostication were assessed (Figure 31.1).

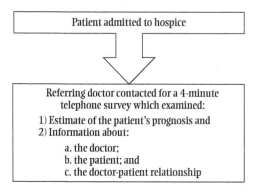

Figure 31.1 Summary of study design.

Study Intervention: Not applicable.

Follow-up: Data were collected through June 30, 1999.

Endpoints: Primary outcome: Observed survival divided by the predicted survival:

- If quotient was between 0.67 and 1.33, prognosis was considered "accurate."
- Quotient less than 0.67 was considered "optimistic" prognostic error.
- Quotient greater than 1.33 was considered "pessimistic" prognostic error.

RESULTS

- Median observed patient survival was 24 days (Table 31.1).

Table 31.1. Factors Associated with Accurate Prognostic Estimate

	n	Optimistic, %[a]	Accurate, %[a]	Pessimistic, %[a]
Disease diagnosis				
Cancer	301	67	20	13
AIDS	58	64	14	22
Others	109	51	22	27
Medical specialties				
Oncology	105	67	23	10
Other medicine subspecialties	79	63	10	27
GIM or geriatric	180	66	17	17
Family practice	67	54	27	19
Surgery or other	30	76	11	13
Median days between last physical examination and outcome of prognostication	—	7.5 days	19.5 days	13.8 days

NOTE: GIM = general internal medicine.

[a]Unless otherwise specified.

- Only 20% of prognoses were accurate.
- Most predictions (63%) were optimistic errors.
- Mean ratio of predicted to observed survival was 5.3.
- Doctors in the upper quartile of practice experience were 63% less likely to make optimistic errors and 78% less likely to make pessimistic errors compared to the average physician.
- Doctors with medical subspecialty training were (excluding oncologists) 3.26 times more likely than geriatricians and general internists to make pessimistic predictions.
- Each additional year that the doctor had known the patient resulted in a 12% increase in the odds of a pessimistic error.
- As the interval since the last physical examination increased, the odds of a doctor making a pessimistic error decreased; each day longer resulted in a 3% decrease in the odds.

Criticisms and Limitations:

- Results may not be generalizable to inpatient hospice programs or hospice programs in other (nonurban) geographic areas.

- The breakdown of diagnoses among patients and medical specialties among doctors in this study may not be generalizable to other hospice programs. In particular, the relatively high prevalence of cancer patients (65%) and relatively low percentage of oncologists (17%) may not be generalizable to other hospices.

Other Relevant Studies and Information:

- The study investigators used a similar prospective cohort to compare physician "formulated" and "communicated" prognoses to terminally ill cancer patients. Physicians reported that they would communicate a frank estimate only 37% of the time and would communicate no estimate, a conscious overestimate, or a conscious underestimate 63% of the time.[2]
- A systematic review found that physicians' clinical prediction of survival (CPS) in terminally ill cancer patients was generally overoptimistic (median CPS 42 days, median actual survival 29 days), overestimating survival by at least 4 weeks 27% of the time.[3]
- A subsequent systematic review of advanced cancer patients' prognostic information preferences showed that all patients wanted honesty from their medical team and the vast majority wanted an indication of their prognosis. Benefits associated with enhanced prognostic awareness included improvements in end-of-life planning.[4]
- Among patients with metastatic solid malignancies and progressive disease, 71% wanted to be told their life expectancy but only 17.6% recalled a prognostic disclosure by their physician, according to a recent study. Prognostic disclosures were associated with more realistic patient expectations of their life expectancy, without adverse effects on patients' emotional well-being or the patient–physician relationship.[5]
- Patients with advanced chemotherapy-refractory cancers whom oncologists expected to die within 6 months had a more accurate understanding of their illnesses following recent discussions of prognosis/life expectancy with their oncologists, according to another study.[6]
- A recent study demonstrated that prognostic scores are more accurate in survival estimation than clinician prediction of survival.[7]

Summary and Implications: This is one of the first studies to examine accuracy of clinician prognostication. Among doctors included in this study, only 20% of prognoses were accurate, with a higher rate of optimistic versus pessimistic predictions. On average, doctors overestimated survival by a factor of 5.3. Prognostic errors were less common among experienced physicians and in situations in which the doctors had less direct contact with the patient (which presumably enabled them to be more objective). Use of prediction algorithms may be more accurate than subjective physician prognostication.

CLINICAL CASE: ESTIMATING A PATIENT'S PROGNOSIS

Case History

A 70-year-old woman with a 2-year history of metastatic lung cancer is admitted to an urban hospice program. According to her referring physician, her Eastern Cooperative Oncology Group performance status is 3. Her referring physician has been practicing medicine for the past 4 years. He is board-certified in general internal medicine. He has known the patient for 4 years, has seen the patient 10 times in the past 3 months, and most recently examined the patient 10 days before hospice admission. The referring physician is asked to estimate the patient's prognosis. Should he consult with another physician before providing his answer?

Suggested Answer

The patient and physician in the case both have baseline characteristics that generally match the profile of patients and physicians included in this study. However, the physician is relatively inexperienced and has had more contact with the patient than the average physician in the study. This study suggests that his inexperience, coupled with his more extensive knowledge of the patient, may lead him to offer an inaccurate prognosis. He should consider consulting with a more experienced colleague who is less familiar with the patient. Perhaps an oncologist would be an appropriate physician with whom the internist could discuss the patient's situation, including the prognosis. After this consultation, the internist may be better equipped to provide a more accurate prognosis. Alternatively, prognostic models may be helpful to improve accuracy.

References

1. Christakis NA, Lamont EB. Extent and determinants of error in doctors' prognoses in terminally ill patients: prospective cohort study. *BMJ*. 2000;320(7233):469–472.
2. Lamont EB, Christakis NA. Prognostic disclosure to patients with cancer near the end of life. *Ann Intern Med*. 2001;134(12):1096–1105.

3. Glare P, Virik K, Jones M, et al. A systematic review of physicians' survival predictions in terminally ill cancer patients. *BMJ*. 2003;327(7408):195–198.

4. Innes S, Payne S. Advanced cancer patients' prognostic information preferences: a review. *Palliat Med*. 2009;23(1):29–39.

5. Enzinger AC, Zhang B, Schrag D, Prigerson HG. Outcomes of prognostic disclosure: associations with prognostic understanding, distress, and relationship with physician among patients with advanced cancer. *J Clin Oncol*. 2015;33(32):3809–3816.

6. Epstein AS, Prigerson HG, O'Reilly EM, Maciejewski PK. Discussions of life expectancy and changes in illness understanding in patients with advanced cancer. *J Clin Oncol*. 2016;34(20):2398–2403.

7. Hui D, Park M, Liu D, Paiva CE, Suh SY, Morita T, Bruera E. Clinician prediction of survival versus the Palliative Prognostic Score: Which approach is more accurate? *Eur J Cancer*. 2016;64:89–95.

32

Prognostic Disclosure to Patients with Advanced Cancer

DAVID HUI

> Physicians report that they do not support frank disclosure for most patients with terminal cancer who request specific prognoses.
>
> —LAMONT ET AL.[1]

Research Question: How often do physicians provide frank survival estimates to patients with advanced cancer when requested?

Funding: Soros Foundation Project on Death in America Faculty Scholars Program, the Robert Wood Johnson Clinical Scholars Program, and the National Institutes of Health.

Year Study Began: 1996.

Year Study Published: 2001.

Study Location: 5 outpatient hospice programs in Chicago, IL.

Who Was Studied: Cancer patients admitted to an outpatient hospice program and their referring physicians.

Who Was Excluded: Patients who declined to participate.

How Many Patients: 326 patients and 258 referring physicians.

Study Overview: Physicians were asked to complete a 4-minute telephone survey about their style for discussing and disclosing prognostic information to their patients. The researchers also assessed for predictors of prognostic disclosure style (Figure 32.1).

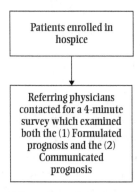

Figure 32.1 Summary of study design.

Study Intervention: Not applicable.

Follow-up: Not applicable.

Endpoints: Prognostic disclosure style was categorized into the following four categories based on the physician's own estimate of patient survival (i.e., formulated prognosis) and what they would tell the patient (i.e., communicated prognosis):

- No disclosure: no communicated prognosis
- Optimistic disclosure: communicated prognosis > formulated prognosis
- Frank disclosure: communicated prognosis = formulated prognosis
- Pessimistic disclosure: communicated prognosis < formulated prognosis

RESULTS

- Among the 412 eligible patients, their physician participated in this study in 326 instances (response rate 79%).
- Almost a quarter of physicians would not communicate a temporally specific prognosis even when asked by patients or families (Table 32.1).

Table 32.1. SUMMARY OF STUDY'S KEY FINDINGS

	No. Patients (%)	Mean Formulated Prognosis (Days)
Physician would not communicate a temporally specific prognosis if asked	68 (23)	92
Physician would communicate a prognosis if asked		
Optimistic disclosure (communicated prognosis > formulated prognosis)	85 (28)	81
Frank disclosure (communicated prognosis = formulated prognosis)	111 (37)	117
Pessimistic disclosure (communicated prognosis < formulated prognosis)	36 (12)	128

- The median actual survival was 26 days; the median formulated prognosis was 75 days (i.e., overestimation in foreseeing); and the median communicated prognosis was 90 days (i.e., overoptimistic in foretelling).
- The formulated prognosis was shorter among the no disclosure and optimistic disclosure groups compared to the frank disclosure and pessimistic disclosure groups (Table 32.1), suggesting that physicians were more likely to avoid disclosure or be overly optimistic when the prognosis was poor.
- Physicians were more likely to have a frank disclosure with older patients and those with lower performance status.
- With regard to physician characteristics, less clinical experience, greater confidence in their formulated prognosis, a practice with fewer patients requiring hospice referral, and male sex were associated with frank disclosure.

Criticisms and Limitations:

- This study was based on survey data involving a hypothetical situation instead of observation of actual care delivery.
- There are other ways of disclosing prognosis, such as using ranges (days, weeks, months). It was unclear if physicians would be more willing to discuss prognostic information if they did not need to provide specific survival times.
- The discrepancy between formulated and communicated prognosis may or may not be intentional, and the reasons for this discrepancy were not examined.

Other Relevant Studies and Information:

- Multiple other studies have demonstrated that clinicians overestimate survival.[2,3]
- The literature also consistently shows that a large proportion of cancer patients either have not had a prognostic discussion or have an inaccurate understanding of their survival.[4]
- An accurate understanding of prognosis is key to decision-making at the end of life.[5,6] Referral to palliative care has also been found to enhance prognostic awareness as well as chemotherapy decisions at the end-of-life.[7]

Summary and Implications: This prospective study highlights that a large proportion of physicians may be reluctant to have a frank prognostic discussion with their patients. Physicians in the study were more likely to withhold prognostic information, or to provide an overly optimistic prognosis, when the prognosis was particularly poor. Because a large portion of patients with advanced illness have an inaccurate understanding of their prognosis, physicians may need more training in the formulation and communication of prognosis.

CLINICAL CASE: HOW TO COMMUNICATE A POOR PROGNOSIS

Case History

A 45-year-old women with metastatic triple negative breast cancer has progressed through multiple lines of palliative systemic therapies and has no further treatment options. Her performance status is 3, and she has lost 15 lbs over the past 3 months. Her oncologist discusses hospice care as an option, and the patient starts crying. She then asks her oncologist, "How long do I have?" Her oncologist believes that her survival is in terms of weeks but hesitates to deliver the bad news.

Suggested Answer

The patient in this case clearly would like to know about her prognosis, which is understandable given how important this information is for end-of-life planning. The literature shows that approximately 80% of cancer patients would like to know about their prognosis, although some patients may be too afraid to ask and would like their doctors to first bring this topic up for discussion.

As demonstrated in this study by Lamont and colleagues, a sizeable proportion of physicians may hesitate to discuss prognosis with their patients even when asked. Potential reasons may include the belief that survival cannot be estimated accurately and/or that the fear that delivery of bad news could take away hope from the patient.

Currently, clinician prediction of survival (i.e., clinical gestate) is often used to formulate a survival estimate. As shown by Lamont et al. as well as others, clinician prediction of survival is often inaccurate and tends to be overly optimistic. Prognostic models that incorporate known prognostic factors (e.g., Palliative Prognostic Index score) have been shown to be more accurate than clinician prediction of survival, and may be useful in this case.

The news may be harsh, but the delivery of it should not be. With proper communication skills training, prognostic discussions can be provided in a sensitive, empathetic, informative fashion. Furthermore, instead of a specific survival time, the oncologist may want to discuss prognosis in terms of general time frames such as "weeks," "months," or even "weeks to months" to highlight the uncertainty in prognostic predictions. This would ensure they are not giving patients an expiry date and that the patient would gain a better understanding of her outlook. A properly conducted prognostic discussion can be an opportunity to empower the patient and family to actively plan ahead.

References

1. Lamont EB, Christakis NA. Prognostic disclosure to patients with cancer near the end of life. *Ann Intern Med.* 2001 Jun 19;134(12):1096–105.
2. Christakis NA, Lamont EB. Extent and determinants of error in doctors' prognoses in terminally ill patients: prospective cohort study. *BMJ.* 2000 Feb 19;320(7233):469–472.
3. Hui D, Kilgore K, Nguyen L, et al. The accuracy of probabilistic versus temporal clinician prediction of survival for patients with advanced cancer: a preliminary report. *Oncologist.* 2011;16(11):1642–1648.
4. Epstein AS, Prigerson HG, O'Reilly EM, Maciejewski PK. Discussions of life expectancy and changes in illness understanding in patients with advanced cancer. *J Clin Oncol.* 2016 May 23. pii: JCO636696. [Epub ahead of print]
5. Weeks JC, Cook EF, O'Day SJ, et al. Relationship between cancer patients' predictions of prognosis and their treatment preferences. *JAMA.* 1998 Jun 3;279(21):1709–1714.

6. Enzinger AC, Zhang B, Schrag D, Prigerson HG. Outcomes of prognostic disclosure: associations with prognostic understanding, distress, and relationship with physician among patients with advanced cancer. *J Clin Oncol*. 2015 Nov 10;33(32):3809–3816.

7. Temel JS, Greer JA, Admane S, et al. Longitudinal perceptions of prognosis and goals of therapy in patients with metastatic non-small-cell lung cancer: results of a randomized study of early palliative care. *J Clin Oncol*. 2011 Jun 10; 29(17):2319–2326.

33

Expectations about Effects of Chemotherapy in Patients with Advanced Cancer

RAJIV AGARWAL AND ANDREW S. EPSTEIN

Patients receiving chemotherapy for incurable cancers may not understand that chemotherapy is unlikely to be curative, which could compromise their ability to make informed treatment decisions that are consonant with their preferences.

—WEEKS ET AL.[1]

Research Question: What are the expectations of patients with incurable cancers about the effectiveness of chemotherapy and likelihood of cure, and what clinical, sociodemographic, and health system factors may be associated with the expectation that chemotherapy might be curative?

Funding: National Cancer Institute.

Year Study Began: 2003.

Year Study Published: 2012.

Study Location: 5 geographic regions (northern California, Los Angeles County, North Carolina, Iowa, and Alabama), 5 large health maintenance organizations, and 15 Veterans Affairs facilities.

Who Was Studied: Adults who were alive 4 months after diagnosis and received chemotherapy for metastatic stage IV lung or colorectal cancer.

Who Was Excluded: Patients with stage I to III or unknown stage, when item on effectiveness of chemotherapy was not asked, and patients who did not receive chemotherapy.

How Many Patients: 1,193.

Study Overview: This is a secondary analysis of collected survey data from the Cancer Care Outcomes Research and Surveillance (CanCORS) national prospective cohort study. The primary aim was to characterize the expectations of patients with stage IV lung or colorectal cancer who opted for chemotherapy treatment about the effectiveness and role of chemotherapy. The researchers also investigated what clinical, sociodemographic, and health system determinants were associated with the belief that receiving chemotherapy may be curative in the metastatic setting (Figure 33.1).

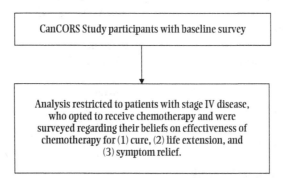

Figure 33.1 Summary of study design.

Baseline surveys were conducted by professional interviewers, who used computer-assisted telephone interview software for administering the surveys and recording responses.

Study Intervention: Not applicable.

Follow-up: Not applicable.

Endpoints: Effectiveness of chemotherapy was assessed with the survey question: "After talking with your doctors about chemotherapy, how likely did you think it was that chemotherapy would . . . help you live longer, cure your cancer, or help you with problems you were having because of cancer?" To identify factors independently associated with inaccurate expectations about the curative potential of chemotherapy, the following variables were analyzed: cancer type, age, gender, educational level, race or ethnic group, marital status, household income, treatment in integrated health care networks, physical function (EQ-5D), patient–physician role in decision-making, and physician communication scores (derived from Consumer Assessment of Healthcare Providers and Systems).[2]

RESULTS

- Among the 1,193 patients eligible for analysis, 69% of those with metastatic lung cancer and 81% of those with metastatic colorectal cancer provided responses that indicated they believed that chemotherapy might be curative (Table 33.1).

Table 33.1. SUMMARY OF STUDY'S KEY FINDINGS

Factors Associated with Expectation of Cure with Chemotherapy	Odds Ratio Relative to Reference (95% CI)	P Value
Cancer Subtype		
Lung (69% cure, n = 710)	Reference	<0.001
Colorectal (81% cure, n = 484)	1.75 (1.29, 2.37)	
Race		
White	Reference	<0.001
Hispanic or Latino	2.82 (1.51, 5.27)	
Black	2.93 (1.80, 4.78)	
Asian/Pacific Islander	4.32 (2.19, 8.49)	
Other	3.07 (1.50, 6.27)	
Integrated Health Care Network		
No	Reference	0.02
Yes	0.70 (0.52, 0.94)	
Physician Communication Score		
Low	Reference	0.002
Intermediate	1.37 (0.93, 2.02)	
High (Perfect Score)	1.90 (1.33, 2.72)	

NOTE: CI = confidence interval.

- Patients with colorectal cancer believed that chemotherapy was more likely to be effective than those with lung cancer. Both groups believed that chemotherapy was more likely to achieve life extension than cure.
- Independent variables associated with inaccurate expectations about the likelihood of cure with chemotherapy included (a) diagnosis

of colorectal cancer compared to lung cancer, (b) non-white race compared to white, (c) not receiving care in an integrated health care network, and (d) paradoxically, higher scores for physician communication (Table 33.1).

- The authors comment that patients who rate their physicians as better communicators may do so when chemotherapy is presented in a more optimistic manner. Alternatively, encounter satisfaction rates and how patients regard physician communication might have been affected by the learning and processing of bad news.
- Education, functional status, income, and patient's role in decision-making were not significantly associated with inaccurate expectations about cure.

Criticisms and Limitations:

- It remains unclear which communication factors in the patient–physician encounter may have influenced a patient's understanding that chemotherapy would offer cure for metastatic disease.
- There may be a difference between what patients hoped for versus what they expected, what they reported versus what they believed, and what they understood versus what they were told. It is possible that these distinctions were not clear in the survey wording.
- The survey was conducted at a single moment in patients' disease courses without longitudinal data, and it is possible that patient responses and comprehension of the realistic goals of chemotherapy could have changed over time.

Other Relevant Studies and Information:

- The objectives and methods of the CanCORS study are described in further detail in the original articles.[3,4] Accurate illness understanding helps patients with advanced cancer make informed decisions.[5] Further studies are needed to determine if improved illness understanding can impact patients' expectations regarding the effectiveness of chemotherapy, as inaccurate perceptions of prognosis are associated with inaccurate belief in curability.[6]
- Findings from Mack et al. further demonstrate that patients with advanced cancer who were well informed about the unlikelihood of cure with chemotherapy received end-of-life chemotherapy at similar rates to those for other patients but were more likely to enroll in hospice before death.[7]

- Fatalism and medical mistrust are more common in minorities with advanced cancer.[8] These could account for some of the differences in expectations of the effectiveness of chemotherapy among non-white racial groups.

Summary and Implications: This analysis of the CanCORS cohort highlights that most patients with stage IV lung or colorectal cancer had inaccurate expectations regarding the curative potential of chemotherapy. Colorectal cancer, non-white race, and high physician communication scores were independently associated with inaccurate expectations. Oncologists may benefit from further training in communication skills related to the benefits and harms of chemotherapy for metastatic cancer.

CLINICAL CASE: WHAT DO PATIENTS EXPECT WITH CHEMOTHERAPY?

Case History

A 55-year-old Hispanic man with newly diagnosed stage IV colorectal adenocarcinoma with liver and lung metastases discusses his chemotherapeutic options with his oncologist. He has a performance status of 1. His oncologist informs him that his disease cannot be cured. The patient expresses understanding and proceeds to ask about the side effects of the chemotherapy. After his oncologist extensively reviews the patient's treatment regimen and logistics, the patient and his wife leave to meet with one of the treatment nurses and comment that they were very satisfied with their encounter. What may this patient expect regarding the effectiveness of chemotherapy and likelihood of cure?

Suggested Answer

As demonstrated in this study by Weeks et al., patients with advanced cancer may inaccurately believe that chemotherapy and other treatments can lead to cure. The patient in this case scenario, due to his race and having advanced colorectal cancer, is at higher risk for this expectation based on the study's findings. Although the oncologist discloses that the patient has metastatic disease that cannot be cured, the patient and his wife may have left the clinic encounter with an overly optimistic view about the effectiveness of chemotherapy. As a result of this fundamental misunderstanding, the patient may not accurately understand the severity of his illness and therefore cannot make truly informed decisions about his treatment. Furthermore, the patient may be satisfied with how his oncologist conveyed information, but this may represent an underlying cognitive processing error, in which the content of the information may be lost if presented in a way that the patient views as favorable. It is important for the oncologist to recognize the clinical, sociodemographic, and health system factors that are associated with the patient's inaccurate hope that cure remains possible. The oncologist may be able to help his patient recognize that treatment is not curative by means of early prognostic discussions, referral to concurrent palliative care, and continuous clinic assessments of the patient's understanding of his illness and goals of chemotherapy.

References

1. Weeks JC, Catalano PJ, Cronin A, et al. Patients' expectations about effects of chemotherapy for advanced cancer. *N Engl J Med*. 2012;367(17):1616–1625.
2. Hays RD, Shaul JA, Williams VS, et al. Psychometric properties of the CAHPS 1.0 survey measures. Consumer Assessment of Health Plans Study. *Med Care*. 1999;37(3 Suppl):Ms22–Ms31.
3. Ayanian JZ, Chrischilles EA, Fletcher RH, et al. Understanding cancer treatment and outcomes: the Cancer Care Outcomes Research and Surveillance Consortium. *J Clin Oncol*. 2004;22(15):2992–2996.
4. Malin JL, Ko C, Ayanian JZ, et al. Understanding cancer patients' experience and outcomes: development and pilot study of the Cancer Care Outcomes Research and Surveillance patient survey. *Support Care Cancer*. 2006;14(8):837–848.
5. Epstein AS, Prigerson HG, O'Reilly EM, et al. Discussions of life expectancy and changes in illness understanding in patients with advanced cancer. *J Clin Oncol*. 2016;34(20):2398–2403.
6. Temel JS, Greer JA, Admane S, et al. Longitudinal perceptions of prognosis and goals of therapy in patients with metastatic non-small-cell lung cancer: results of a randomized study of early palliative care. *J Clin Oncol*. 2011;29(17):2319–2326.
7. Mack JW, Walling A, Dy S, et al. Patient beliefs that chemotherapy may be curative and care received at the end of life among patients with metastatic lung and colorectal cancer. *Cancer*. 2015;121(11):1891–1897.
8. Bergamo C, Lin JJ, Smith C, et al. Evaluating beliefs associated with late-stage lung cancer presentation in minorities. *J Thorac Oncol*. 2013;8(1):12–18.

34

Physician Message and Patient's Perception of Compassion

LYNN A. FLINT AND ERIC WIDERA

> In this randomized clinical trial, we found that physicians delivering a more optimistic message were perceived as more compassionate as compared with equally empathetic physicians delivering a less optimistic message.
>
> —TANCO ET AL.[1]

Research Question: Do patients perceive physicians delivering an optimistic message as more compassionate than those delivering a less optimistic but more realistic message?

Funding: Department of Palliative Care and Rehabilitation Medicine, University of Texas MD Anderson Cancer Center.

Year Study Began: 2013.

Year Study Published: 2015.

Study Location: Supportive Care Center in MD Anderson Cancer Center, Houston, TX.

Who Was Studied: English-speaking adults aged 18 or older with advanced cancer, defined as locally advanced, recurrent, or metastatic.

Who Was Excluded: Patients with cognitive impairment and/or severe physical or emotional symptoms interfering with their ability to participate in the study as determined by the attending palliative care physician or the principal investigator.

How Many Patients: 100.

Study Overview: See Figure 34.1 for a summary of the study design.

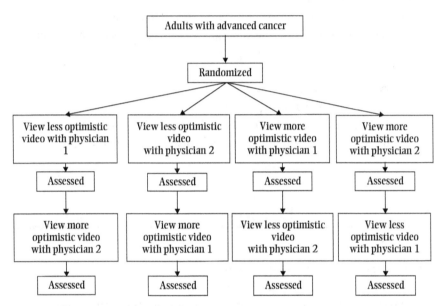

Figure 34.1 Summary of study design.

Study Intervention: Participants watched videos of professional actors playing a patient and physician discussing cancer treatment and prognosis. The researchers produced four videos depicting a patient with advanced cancer and functional decline who is not a good candidate for further cancer-directed therapy. Two different actors (physician 1 and physician 2) with similar demographics portrayed the physician. They displayed the same number of empathic behaviors in each video.

Two different scripts were used. In the "less optimistic" script, the physician provided clear information about the lack of further treatment options. In the "more optimistic" script, the physician discussed the possibility of more treatment if the patient's performance status improved. Each script was recorded with both physician 1 and physician 2 (four videos in total).

Each participant was randomized to watch two videos (Figure 34.1). This crossover design allowed for intraindividual comparison and patient preference to be elicited.

Follow-up: Participants' perceptions were assessed using a variety of survey measures immediately after viewing each video. Physician compassion was measured after each video.

Endpoints:

Primary outcome measure:
- Patient rating of physician compassion using a tool assessing 5 dimensions: warm/cold, pleasant/unpleasant, compassionate/distant, sensitive/insensitive, and caring/uncaring

Secondary outcome measures:
- Patient-reported physician preference
- Patient rating of physician professionalism including assessment of patients' perceptions of the physicians' trustworthiness and ability to provide care

RESULTS

Patient characteristics/baseline measures:
- Median age 57, 52% female, 76% white
- No significant difference in preference for a more optimistic message or more realistic message before watching videos

Primary outcomes:
- After viewing just the first video, participants rated the physicians with the more optimistic message as significantly more compassionate than the physician with the less optimistic message.
- After viewing both videos, participants rated the physician in the second video as more compassionate than the physician in the first video in all four arms.
- Overall, after viewing both videos, participants rated the physicians with the more optimistic message as more compassionate than those with the less optimistic message.

Secondary outcomes:
- After viewing both videos, more participants preferred the physician in the second video viewed (second-order effect).
- The majority (57%) of patients preferred the physician delivering the more optimistic message.
- After viewing both videos, participants perceived the physician with the more optimistic message to be more trustworthy and more able to provide care.
- In multivariate analysis, degree of trust, video sequence, and type of message were associated with rating of physician compassion, with patients who reported greater degree of trust in the health care system reporting greater perceptions of compassion.

Criticisms and Limitations:

- A video study offers an artificial environment in which study participants may consider themselves to be "spectators" instead of "patients."
- Factors other than the content of the message, such as body language, may have influenced participants' ratings of compassion. The authors did not bring in external experts in nonverbal communication to review the videos to assess for this possibility.
- This study examines only one message (no more treatment vs. more treatment may be possible). It is unclear if the communication of other types of bad news (e.g., prognosis, hospice referral) may have a similar impact.

Other Relevant Studies and Information:

- Other studies have demonstrated a relationship between optimistic physician messages and better patient perceptions of physicians. For example, patients receiving palliative chemotherapy who believed there was a chance the treatment could be curative were more likely to rate their physicians' communication skills favorably than those who did not believe treatment could lead to cure.[2]
- In a qualitative study of transcripts from oncology visits with patients with advanced cancer, pessimistic communication was shown to be associated with a more accurate patient report of a poor prognosis, whereas optimistic communication had no relationship with the accuracy of patient-reported prognosis.[3]

- In another study, surrogates of intensive care patients were asked to interpret a range of hypothetical prognostic statements. A majority of surrogates interpreted pessimistic prognostic statements optimistically, but they did not interpret optimistic prognostic statements pessimistically.[4] Other studies have shown an association between realistic prognostic disclosure and more realistic patient estimate of life expectancy without worsening anxiety, depression, or physician–patient relationship.[5]

Summary and Implications: This study found that patients with advanced cancer rated physicians delivering a more optimistic message in video scenarios as more compassionate than those delivering a less optimistic message. It represents one of the key studies to nicely illustrate the difficult balance between fostering realistic hope and running the risk of negatively affecting the patient-clinician relationship.

CLINICAL CASE: WOULD YOU DELIVER BAD NEWS TO THIS PATIENT?

Case History

A 57-year-old man with unresectable pancreatic cancer has an appointment with his oncologist to discuss the results of his recent CT scan after several cycles of palliative chemotherapy. The patient reported to the nurse that he has been more fatigued lately and is spending most of his day in bed or a chair. The scan shows increase in size of the pancreatic mass and new liver metastases. The oncologist believes that further chemotherapy would be harmful, but she is unsure how to break this news to the patient and his wife. The oncologist highly values her relationship with the patient and family. She wants them to trust her and to know that she cares deeply about them, particularly as they look toward a difficult future path. She is also aware that her hospital is now measuring patient satisfaction ratings, and they are testing new quality measures focused on patient–physician communication. Should she deliver the bad news and inform them today that further treatments are not available? Or should she deliver the bad news and tell them that he might be eligible for further treatment in the future if he becomes stronger?

Suggested Answer

She should ask her patient and his wife about their preferences for information, ask permission to speak about some difficult news, and, if desired, inform them of the results of the CT scan in plain language, avoiding medical jargon. She recognizes that they may not be able to absorb more information today and offers a second appointment to review the results and next steps. They ask about treatment options and she says that, although she wishes things were different, he is not a candidate for further cancer-directed therapy. She reaffirms her ongoing commitment to help ease his symptoms and to continue to care for him.

References

1. Tanco K, Rhondall W, Perez-Cruz P, et al. Patient perception of physician compassion after a more optimistic vs a less optimistic message: a randomized clinical trial. *JAMA Oncol.* 2015(2):176–183.
2. Weeks, JC, Cook F, O'Day SJ, et al. Relationship between cancer patients' predictions of prognosis and their treatment preferences. *JAMA.* 1998;279:1709–1714.
3. Robinson, TM, Alexander, SC, Hays M, et al. Patient-oncologist communication in advanced cancer: predictors of patient perception of prognosis. *Support Care Cancer.* 2008;16:1049–1057.
4. Zier LS, Sottile PD, Hong SY, Weissfield LA, White DB. Surrogate decision-makers' interpretation of prognostic information: a mixed methods study. *Ann Intern Med.* 2012;156:360–366.
5. Enzinger AC, Zhang B, Schrag D, Prigerson HG. Outcomes of prognostic disclosure: associations with prognostic understanding, distress, and relationship with physician among patients with advanced cancer. *J Clin Oncol.* 2015;33(32):3809–3816.

End of Life Care and Planning

35

Association Between Advance Directives and Quality of End-of-Life Care

DONNA S. ZHUKOVSKY

> Bereaved family member report of completion of an AD was associated with greater use of hospice and fewer reported concerns with communication, yet important opportunities remain to improve the quality of end-of-life care.
>
> —TENO ET AL.[1]

Research Question: What is the association between the presence of written advance directives (ADs) and quality of end-of-life (EOL) care?

Funding: Robert Wood Johnson Foundation (Grant 037188).

Year Study Began: 2000.

Year Study Published: 2007.

Study Location: United States.

Who Was Studied: Adults who died of a nontraumatic cause in the hospital, at home, or in nursing homes in the year 2000.

Who Was Excluded: People who died of traumatic causes and children.

How Many Patients: 1,553 (reported on by 1,553 family surrogates).

Study Overview: See Figure 35.1 for a summary of the study design.

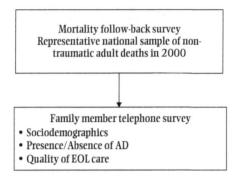

Figure 35.1 Mortality follow-back survey study schema.

Study Intervention: Telephone interviews were conducted with a representative sample of family members of people who had died of nontraumatic causes in the year 2000. Most interviews were conducted 9 to 15 months postmortem. Family members were asked if the person had a written AD.

Measures of quality of EOL care across 5 domains were derived from qualitative review of professional guidelines, consumer focus groups, and experts.[2] These included

1. Desired level of physical comfort and emotional comfort received (3 items)
2. Promotion of shared decision-making (3 items)
3. Respectful treatment of patient (1 item)
4. Coordination of care (1 item)
5. Family's need for information (3 items)

The tool also contains a summary assessment, calculated as the sum of domain scores (0–50, higher is better).[3,4]

A multivariate logistic regression analysis was conducted to evaluate the association between each domain and AD completion, adjusted for age, race/ethnicity, underlying cause of death, respondent perceptions of if death expected, and if decedent had difficulty raising from bed or chair 90 days before death.

Follow-up: Not applicable.

Endpoints: The association between the presence of written ADs and
1. Family perception of quality of EOL care in the last month of life
2. Last place of care

RESULTS

- 71% of decedents were reported to have at least one AD by family members (Table 35.1).

Table 35.1. SUMMARY OF STUDY'S KEY FINDINGS

	Advance Directive Reported	No Advance Directive Reported	P Value
Sample Size, actual (weighted)	1,130 (1,367,560)	423 (565,632)	
Last place of care			<0.001
Home + visiting nurse	12.3%	20.04%	
Home with hospice	18.5%	10.1%	
Nursing home	35.2%	20.3%	
Hospital	34.0%	49.2%	
Died in ICU	11.8%	22.0%	0.002
Respirator: last month	25.6%	36.7%	0.005
Feeding Tube: last month	17.3%	26.8%	0.002
Specific wishes for care	72.4%	32.1%	0.002
Wishes discussed with provider	74.4%	68.6%	0.31
Care inconsistent with wishes	9.7%	9.5%	0.97
Insufficient help with:			**Adjusted Relative Risk (95% confidence interval)**
Pain	23.4	28.3	1.2 (0.7–1.9)
Dyspnea	21.8	24.3	1.0 (0.7–1.3)
Emotional support	47.6	57.1	0.9 (0.7–1.1)
Concerns with provider communication about decision-making	19.7	32.2	1.4 (1.1–1.6)
Insufficient communication about dying process	39.4	53.6	1.2 (1.0–1.3)

NOTE: ICU = intensive care unit.

- Decedents reported to have ADs versus those without an AD were more likely to be older, female, and white; to have higher educational level; to be unmarried; and to have a cancer diagnosis. Those with an AD were also less likely to die an unexpected death.
- Individuals reported to have ADs were more likely to die in a nursing home or at home with hospice than in hospital ($P < 0.001$) and less likely to die in an intensive care unit ($P = 0.002$).
- As compared to people without a written AD, individuals reported to have an AD were less likely to receive mechanical ventilation (25.6% vs. 36.7%; $P = 0.005$) or use feeding tubes in the last month of life (17.3% vs. 26.8%; $P = 0.002$). There was no statistical difference in mean number of days spent in hospice care (48.7 vs. 59.3; $P = 0.55$).
- Decedents reported to have ADs were more likely to have communicated specific wishes for their care than individuals without ADs (72.4% vs. 32.1%; $P = 0.002$). However, for individuals who had expressed wishes, there was no significant difference in communication of those wishes to physicians, regardless of AD status (74.4% vs. 68.8%; $P = 0.31$) or in receipt of care inconsistent with their wishes (9.7% vs. 9.5%; $P = 0.97$).
- Decedents with ADs were not reported to experience major differences in quality of EOL care, with the exception of higher rates of shared decision-making and family preparation for death.
- Despite family endorsement of relatively high levels of EOL care, multiple unmet needs were apparent from survey responses.

Criticisms and Limitations:

- The After Death Bereaved Family Member Interview has undergone preliminary but incomplete validation.[3,4]
- Due to the choice of study methodology, outcome measures relied on surrogate reports of patient reported outcomes, compounded by the bias implicit in retrospective recall.
- Family reports of written ADs as a surrogate for advance care planning may not adequately represent the advance care planning process. More specifically, the presence of ADs does not reflect the extent to which the person has reflected on future care options through the lens of his or her values and communicated those preferences to key stakeholders involved in his or her care.[5]
- The largely negative outcomes between groups with respect to association with quality of EOL care may relate to individuals who

completed documents without a comprehensive understanding of care options or in-depth evaluation of values and goals for care. In contrast, the lack of significant difference in care received among those with expressed wishes for care, regardless of AD status, suggests that some individuals engaged in advance care planning without completing or sharing ADs.

Other Relevant Studies and Information:

- ADs are frequently used as a marker for the advance care planning process. Advance care planning interventions are known to increase completion of ADs and, when they include discussion of EOL, improve the congruence of care preferred with care the person received.[6] However, to date, incorporating patient, family, and health care provider reports as outcomes, such as of advance care planning interventions, is relatively infrequent at the systems level.[7]
- The frequency of advance directives is surprisingly high, as compared to other national surveys.[8,9] The study under review represents a sample "enriched" with individuals who had chronic illness and were older and thus more likely to have completed ADs.

Summary and Implications: This study demonstrates that patients with ADs are more likely to have specific wishes for care and that completion of ADs was associated with less aggressive care in the last month of life (e.g., hospital death, intensive care unit death, mechanical ventilation feeding tube). Additional research evaluating the impact of different components of the advance care planning process on care outcomes and with patients and family satisfaction with care is needed.

CLINICAL CASE: HOW TO ASCERTAIN PATIENT PREFERENCES FOR END-OF-LIFE CARE

Case History

You are a geriatrician who is asked to consult on the care of a frail 79-year-old woman, Mrs. W, with mild dementia. She has just moved to your community to live with her daughter after having been recently widowed. Her daughter, who accompanies her to the visit, asks you to discuss different living arrangements and care options, should the patient deteriorate. She does not know if her mother has any advance directives. How might you approach the situation?

Suggested Answer

How to approach the situation will in part depend on the extent to which the patient's dementia limits her participation in the discussion. Because her dementia is mild, she may well be able to be a full partner in the advance care planning process. After spending some time getting to know Mrs. W and establishing rapport, you can start by asking her if she is open to discussion about her medical care in the future, should she become weaker and more ill. If she is agreeable, you may be able to draw on her experience with her husband's care prior to his death or from her knowledge of or experience with other friends or family members to elicit her values and goals for medical decision-making. You can also ask her if she has ever discussed these kinds of things before and, if so, with whom and if she has completed any advance directive documents.

For advance care planning discussions, it is considered best practice to start with her understanding of her medical and life circumstances. In this manner, you can clarify her medical circumstances and provide any needed information. While there is no set format, a next step might be to explore what values and goals direct her care choices. This often simplifies the discussion of what quality of life means to her and what circumstances she would not consider to be acceptable. If she is willing and able, other topics for discussion include who she would like to take care of her if she needs more help, where she would like to be cared for when more ill, and her preferences regarding life-sustaining interventions. For many people, it is hard to decide about future care for a situation they have not yet encountered, so ascertaining what drives their care preferences can prepare them and their family members/proxies for decision-making, when the time gets closer.

If she is not able to or not willing to discuss, she may still be able to indicate who she would like to make medical decisions on her behalf, should the situation arise. With her permission, you can then explore her daughter's knowledge of what values and goals drive her mother's care choices and any previously expressed wishes for care, in a manner similar to that detailed earlier. It is important to keep in mind that the advance care planning process may take more than one session, respecting where the individual is in the advance care planning process and to allow time for reflection with self and family. It is also important to emphasize the need for periodic review of previously established plans, to ensure that they remain pertinent to the person's current life situation.

References

1. Teno JM, Gruneir A, Schwartz Z, Nanda A, Wetle T. Association between advance directives and quality of end-of-life care: a national study. *J Am Geriatr Soc.* 2007;55:189–194.

2. Teno JM, Casey VA, Welch LC, Edgman-Levitan S. Patient-focused, family-centered end-of-life medical care: views of the guidelines and bereaved family members. *J Pain Symptom Manage.* 2001;22:738–751.

3. Teno JM, Clarridge B, Casey V, Edgman-Levitan S, Fowler J. Validation of Toolkit After-Death Bereaved Family Member Interview. *J Pain Symptom Manage.* 2001; 22:752–758.

4. TIME: Toolkit of Instruments to Measure End-of-Life Care. October 1, 2000. Updated February 17, 2004. Retrieved from http://www.chcr.brown.edu/pcoc/

5. Sudore RL, Fried TR. Redefining the "planning" in advance care planning: preparing for end-of-life decision making. *Ann Intern Med.* 2010;153:256–261.

6. Houben CH, Spruit MA, Groenen MT, Wouters EF, Janssen DJ. Efficacy of advance care planning: a systematic review and meta-analysis. *J Am Med Dir Assoc.* 2014;15:477–489.

7. Biondo PD, Lee LD, Davison SN, Simon JE, Advance Care Planning Collaborative Research and Innovation Opportunities Program. How healthcare systems evaluate their advance care planning initiatives: results from a systematic review. *Palliat Med.* 2016;30:720–729.

8. Rao JK, Anderson LA, Lin FC, Laux JP. Completion of advance directives among U.S. consumers. *Am J Prev Med.* 2014;46:65–70.

9. Jones AL, Moss AJ, Harris-Kojetin LD. Use of advance directives in long-term care populations. *NCHS Data Brief.* 2011;54:1–8.

36

Outcomes Associated with End-of-Life Discussions

MASANORI MORI

> Given the adverse outcomes associated with not having end-of-life discussions, there appears to be a need to increase the frequency of these conversations.
>
> —WRIGHT ET AL.[1]

Research Question: Are end-of-life discussions (EOLds) between patients with advanced cancer and their physicians associated with aggressive interventions, patients' psychological distress, quality of life near death, and caregivers' bereavement outcomes?

Funding: Grants CA 106370 from the National Cancer Institute and MH63892 from the National Institute of Mental Health.

Year Study Began: 2002.

Year Study Published: 2008.

Study Location: 7 different outpatient sites in the United States.

Who Was Studied: Patients with advanced cancer (presence of distant metastases and disease refractory to first-line chemotherapy) who had an informal caregiver.

Who Was Excluded: Patient–caregiver dyads in which either the patient or caregiver refused to participate, met criteria for dementia or delirium, or did not speak either English or Spanish were excluded.

How Many Patients: 332.

Study Overview: Coping with Cancer Study was a prospective, longitudinal multisite cohort study of advanced cancer patients and their informal caregivers (Figure 36.1).

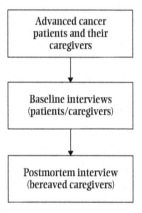

Figure 36.1 Summary of study design.

Patients were followed up from enrollment to death, a median of 4.4 months later. Presence or absence of EOLds was assessed by the question in the baseline interview: "Have you and your doctor discussed any particular wishes you have about the care you would want to receive if you were dying?" Bereaved caregivers' psychiatric illness and quality of life was assessed a median of 6.5 months later.

Study Intervention: Not applicable.

Follow-up: Until death and postmortem interview during the bereavement period.

Endpoints: Medical care at the end of life (intensive care unit [ICU] admission, ventilator use, resuscitation, chemotherapy, feeding tube, outpatient hospice use, and length of time in hospice); mental health (the Structured Clinical Interview for DSM-IV [SCID], the Endicott Scale, and McGill Quality of Life psychological subscale); treatment preferences; advance care planning; patients' quality of life at the end of life (0–10); and bereavement outcomes (SCID, Medical Outcome Study 36-item Short Form Survey, satisfaction and regrets about patient's end-of-life care).

RESULTS

- The cohort consisted of 332 advanced cancer patients who died a median of 4.4 months after enrollment. Overall, 123 of 332 (37.0%) patients reported having EOLds with their physicians at baseline.
- EOLds were not associated with higher rates of mental disorders (e.g., major depressive disorder, generalized anxiety disorder, panic disorder, posttraumatic stress disorder) or more worry or sadness (Table 36.1).
- Patients who reported having EOLds were significantly more likely to accept that their illness was terminal and prefer medical treatment focused on relieving pain and discomfort versus life-extending therapies. They were also more likely to have completed a do-not-resuscitate order (Table 36.1).
- After propensity-score weighted adjustment, EOLds were associated with lower rates of ventilation, resuscitation, ICU admission, and earlier hospice enrollment (Table 36.1).
- In adjusted analyses, more aggressive medical care was associated with worse quality of life in patients (6.4 vs. 4.6; $F = 3.61$, $P = 0.01$), and higher risk of major depressive disorder (adjusted odds ratio [OR] 3.37; 95% confidence interval [CI] 1.12–10.13), regret ($\beta = 0.17$; $P = 0.01$), and unpreparedness for the patient's death ($\beta = -0.30$; $P < 0.001$) in bereaved caregivers. Conversely, longer hospice stays were associated with better patient quality of life (mean score, 6.9 vs. 5.6; $F = 3.70$, $P = 0.01$), compared with a week or less of hospice services.
- Better patient quality of life was associated with better caregiver outcomes, including overall quality of life ($\beta = 0.20$; $P = 0.001$), self-reported health ($\beta = 0.17$, $P = 0.004$), physical functioning ($\beta = 0.14$, $P = 0.02$), mental health ($\beta = 0.13$, $P = 0.04$), and improvements in self-rated change in health (adjusted OR 1.17; 95% CI 1.05–1.29).
- Caregivers of patients with high quality of life at the end of life felt better prepared for the death ($\beta = 0.23$, $P = 0.002$) and experienced less regret ($\beta = -0.30$, $P < 0.001$) at follow-up.

Table 36.1. Associations Between Advanced Cancer Patients' EOLds and End-of-Life Outcomes

	No. (%) Total (N = 332)	End-of-Life Discussion		Adjusted OR (95% Confidence Interval)[a]	P Value
		Yes (n = 123)	No (n = 209)		
Acceptance, preferences, and planning					
Accepts illness is terminal	125 (37.7)	65 (52.9)	60 (28.7)	2.19 (1.40–3.43)	<0.001
Wants to know life expectancy	242 (72.9)	103 (83.7)	139 (66.5)	2.40 (1.43–4.04)	<0.001
Values comfort over life extension	245 (73.8)	105 (85.4)	140 (70.0)	2.63 (1.54–4.49)	<0.001
Against death in ICU	118 (35.5)	60 (48.8)	58 (27.8)	2.13 (1.35–3.37)	<0.001
Completed DNR order	134 (41.1)	75 (63.0)	59 (28.5)	3.12 (1.98–4.90)	<0.001
Completed living will, durable power of attorney, or health care proxy	181 (55.2)	86 (71.7)	95 (46.1)	1.96 (1.25–3.07)	0.003
Medical care received in the last week	332	123 (37.0)	209 (63.0)		
ICU admission	31 (9.3)	5 (4.1)	26 (12.4)	0.35 (0.14–0.90)	0.02
Ventilator use	25 (7.5)	2 (1.6)	23 (11.0)	0.26 (0.08–0.83)	0.02
Resuscitation	15 (4.5)	1 (0.8)	14 (6.7)	0.16 (0.03–0.80)	0.02
Chemotherapy	19 (5.7)	5 (4.1)	14 (6.7)	0.36 (0.13–1.03)	0.08
Feeding tube	26 (7.9)	11 (8.9)	15 (7.3)	1.30 (0.55–3.10)	0.52
Outpatient hospice used	213 (64.4)	93 (76.2)	120 (57.4)	1.50 (0.91–2.48)	0.10
Outpatient hospice ≥1 wk	173 (52.3)	80 (65.6)	93 (44.5)	1.65 (1.04–2.63)	0.03

NOTE: EOLds = end-of-life discussions; DNR = do not resuscitate; ICU = intensive care unit; OR = odds ratio.

[a] The propensity-score weighted sample was used for these analyses.

Criticisms and Limitations:

- The presence or absence of EOLds was assessed based on a single question, "Have you and your doctor discussed any particular wishes you have about the care you would want to receive if you were dying?" which may be oversimplified and subject to recall bias.
- Detailed information about the EOLd, including its depth and quality, were not examined.
- Because this was an observational study, one cannot make causal inferences about outcomes.
- Propensity-score weighting could not correct for unmeasured or hidden biases.
- As end-of-life conversations can be markedly influenced by cultures, one should take caution when applying these findings to patients of other cultural backgrounds or in different countries.

Other Relevant Studies and Information:

- Both the Coping with Cancer Study and the CANCORs study found that EOLds are associated with the receipt of care consistent with patients' preferences and that early EOLds are prospectively associated with less aggressive care and greater use of hospice at EOL.[2,3]
- Many EOLds in advanced cancer patients occur during acute hospital care, with providers other than oncologists and late in the course of illness. Physicians' discomfort talking about death, lower physician-perceived importance of autonomy, and life completion in experiencing a good death have been shown to be barriers to timely discussions.[4–6]
- Multiple barriers to effective EOLds associated with patients, caregivers, clinicians, and systems have been identified. Multifaceted interventions to effective EOLds are thus needed.[7]

Summary and Implications: This study is one of the first to convincingly demonstrate that EOLds are associated with improved outcomes in patients and bereaved caregivers, as well as less aggressive medical care near death and earlier hospice referrals. It also showed that the benefits among patients with advanced cancer and their families were achieved without associated increased rates of emotional distress or psychiatric disorders.

These findings may help destigmatize EOLds and assist physicians and patients in initiating such conversations and engaging in advance care planning.

CLINICAL CASE: SHOULD A PHYSICIAN HAVE END-OF-LIFE DISCUSSIONS WITH THIS PATIENT?

Case History

A 55-year-old woman with metastatic pancreatic cancer has progressed through the first line of chemotherapy. Today she visits her oncologist's office with her husband to discuss the next treatment options. Her general condition is relatively stable with performance status of 1. As a manager of a large company and mother of two college students, she has always planned ahead in her work and personal life. After detailed discussions on potentially limited benefits and side effects of the next chemotherapy options, she asks you what if the treatment did not work and what she should keep in mind to plan ahead.

Suggested Answer

Multiple studies including the one reported here showed cascading benefits of early EOLds in patients and their families. The oncologist can apply these findings in this case of a patient with advanced pancreatic cancer and limited life expectancy. The patient clearly indicates that she is prepared to discuss what she should consider for the future.

Thus the oncologist may want to ask about the patient's understanding of her disease and prognosis and explore her wishes, goals, and preferences of future care she would want to receive if there were no more standard treatment to offer and she were dying. Such conversations may occur in a single visit or over several encounters. During the discussions, the oncologist may want to reassure the patient and her husband that whatever treatment options she chooses, and however that develops, he will continue to respect her wishes and take good care of her.

References

1. Wright AA, Zhang B, Ray A, et al. Associations between end-of-life discussions, patient mental health, medical care near death, and caregiver bereavement adjustment. *JAMA*. 2008 Oct 8;300(14):1665–1673.
2. Mack JW, Weeks JC, Wright AA, Block SD, Prigerson HG. End-of-life discussions, goal attainment, and distress at the end of life: predictors and outcomes of receipt of care consistent with preferences. *J Clin Oncol*. 2010 Mar 1;28(7):1203–1208.
3. Mack JW, Cronin A, Keating NL, et al. Associations between end-of-life discussion characteristics and care received near death: a prospective cohort study. *J Clin Oncol*. 2012 Dec 10;30(35):4387–4395.

4. Mack JW, Cronin A, Taback N, et al. End-of-life care discussions among patients with advanced cancer: a cohort study. *Ann Intern Med.* 2012 Feb 7;156(3):204–210.

5. Keating NL, Landrum MB, Rogers SO Jr, et al. Physician factors associated with discussions about end-of-life care. *Cancer.* 2010 Feb 15;116(4):998–1006.

6. Mori M, Shimizu C, Ogawa A, Okusaka T, Yoshida S, Morita T. A National survey to systematically identify factors associated with oncologists' attitudes toward end-of-life discussions: What determines timing of end-of-life discussions? *Oncologist.* 2015 Nov;20(11):1304–1311.

7. Bernacki RE, Block SD, American College of Physicians High Value Care Task Force. Communication about serious illness care goals: a review and synthesis of best practices. *JAMA Intern Med.* 2014 Dec;174(12):1994–2003.

37

End-of-Life Discussions and Aggressiveness of Care Received Near Death

YAEL SCHENKER AND JUSTIN YU

> We found that patients [with advanced cancer] who had earlier discussions about EOL care were less likely to receive aggressive measures before death.
>
> —MACK ET AL.[1]

Research Question: What is the relationship between end-of-life (EOL) discussion characteristics (timing, location, and involved providers) and the aggressiveness of medical care received near death in patients with advanced cancer?

Funding: National Cancer Institute, Department of Veterans Affairs, American Cancer Society, National Palliative Care Research Center.

Year Study Began: 2003.

Year Study Published: 2012.

Study Location: Northern California, Los Angeles County, North Carolina, Iowa, and Alabama, or patients received care in one of five large HMOs or one of 15 VA sites included in CanCORS study.[2]

Who Was Studied: Patients with stage IV lung or colorectal cancer at diagnosis enrolled in the prospective CanCORS Cohort.

Who Was Excluded: Patients/surrogates who declined to participate, stage I to III cancer at diagnosis, medical records were unavailable, died within 1 month of diagnosis, and/or survived to the end of the 15-month medical record abstraction period.

How Many Patients: 1,231.

Study Overview: This prospective cohort study interviewed patients (or surrogates for patients who were deceased or too ill to participate) *and* abstracted their pertinent medical records. Information was collected on the presence/absence of EOL discussion, discussion characteristics (timing, involved providers, and location), and type of EOL care received (Figure 37.1).

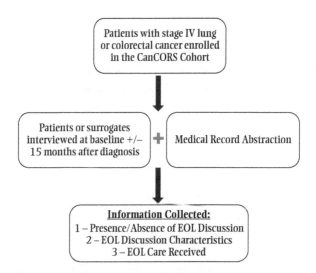

Figure 37.1 Summary of study design.

Study Intervention: Not applicable.

Follow-up: Death or up to 15 months after diagnosis.

Endpoints: Markers of aggressive EOL care: chemotherapy in the last 14 days of life, acute care in last 30 days of life (>1 emergency department visit/hospitalization or >14-day hospitalization), intensive care unit (ICU) care in last 30 days of life, and hospice initiation in the last 7 days of life.

RESULTS

- Of the 1,231 patients studied, 82% (n = 1,009) had lung cancer and 18% (n = 222) had colorectal cancer.
- 88% (1,082) of patients had EOL discussions documented.
  - 48% of these patients had discussions reported in both medical records and during patient/surrogate interviews.
  - 17% had discussions reported in medical records only.
  - 23% had discussions reported in patient or surrogate interviews only.
- Of the *initial EOL discussions* documented in the medical records:
  - 39% occurred in last 30 days of life.
  - 63% occurred in an acute hospital setting.
  - 40% included oncologists.
- Overall, 16% of patients received chemotherapy in the last 14 days of life, 40% received acute care in the last 30 days of life, and 6% received ICU care in the last 30 days of life. In adjusted analysis, EOL discussions reported by patients or surrogates, especially if performed early (more than 30 days before death), were associated with significantly less aggressive EOL care. Discussions documented in the medical record only (without patient or surrogate report) were not associated with less aggressive care (Tables 37.1 and 37.2).
- Initial EOL discussion performed >30 days prior to death was also associated with decreased likelihood of initiating hospice within 7 days of death.
- Patients who had initial EOL discussions in the hospital setting were more likely to receive acute care (odds ratio [OR] 3.06, 95% confidence interval [CI] 2.29–4.1) and ICU care (OR 2.77, 95% CI 1.56–4.91) in the last 30 days of life, and initiate hospice within the last week of life (OR 3.43, 95% CI 2.08–5.64).

Table 37.1. Presence of EOL Discussion and EOL Care Received

Presence of EOL Discussion	Any Aggressive Care		Chemotherapy in Last 14 DOL		Acute Care in Last 30 DOL		ICU Care in Last 30 DOL	
	OR	95% CI	OR	95% CI	OR	95% CI	OR	95% CI
No	Reference							
Medical record only	1.13	0.68–1.89	0.81	0.44–1.48	1.16	0.7–1.91	2.02	0.78–5.23
Interview +/− medical record	0.40	0.27–0.60	0.41	0.25–0.66	0.43	0.29–0.65	0.77	0.33–1.80

NOTE: EOL = end of life; DOL = days of life; ICU = intensive care unit; OR = odds ratio; CI = confidence interval.

Table 37.2. Timing of EOL Discussion and EOL Care Received

Days Between First EOL Discussion and Death	Any Aggressive Care		Chemotherapy in Last 14 DOL		Acute Care in Last 30 DOL		ICU Care in Last 30 DOL	
	OR	95% CI	OR	95% CI	OR	95% CI	OR	95% CI
≤30	Reference							
31–60	0.52	0.36–0.76	0.42	0.24–0.74	0.65	0.44–0.94	0.65	0.31–1.35
61–90	0.38	0.24–0.61	0.38	0.18–0.80	0.44	0.27–0.71	0.69	0.28–1.69
>90	0.46	0.31–0.68	0.74	0.43–1.25	0.42	0.28–0.64	0.37	0.14–0.95

NOTE: These results were calculated with adjusted analyses. EOL = end of life; DOL = days of life; OR = odds ratio; CI = confidence interval.

Criticisms and Limitations:

- This study included only patients with stage IV cancer at diagnosis and excluded patients with stage I to III disease, who might have progressed to advanced disease.
- The majority of patients who were studied had lung cancer (82%).
- Patients who lived longer than 15 months after diagnosis of stage IV cancer were excluded.
- This study did not attempt to evaluate the content or quality of EOL discussion.

Other Relevant Studies and Information:

- Prior studies have shown that when patients with advanced cancer have EOL discussions with their physicians, they receive EOL care that is less aggressive and more consistent with their stated preferences.[3,4]
- Multiple national oncologic society guidelines recommend that EOL conversations between patients with advanced cancer and their physicians occur soon after diagnosis.[5,6]
- The CanCORS study also found that a majority of patients with metastatic lung and gastrointestinal cancer patients believed that their disease is potentially curable.[7] More recently, it reported that aggressive measures, such as ICU deaths, were associated with worse quality of end-of-life care as perceived by bereaved caregivers.[8]

Summary and Implications: This prospective study demonstrated that a significant proportion of patients with advanced cancer do not have a discussion about EOL care until they are clinically deteriorating (last month of life and/or hospitalized). Importantly, it also showed that patients who reported having an EOL discussion with their providers were less likely to receive aggressive EOL care. This was especially true if these discussion occurred earlier (>30 days between discussion and death) and outside the inpatient hospital setting. Therefore physicians who treat patients with advanced cancer should consider initiating EOL conversations closer to the time of diagnosis, "while the patient is doing comparatively well, [and] has time to plan."[1]

CLINICAL CASE: WHEN SHOULD PHYSICIANS INITIATE DISCUSSIONS ABOUT END-OF-LIFE CARE?

Case History

A 67-year-old man has been diagnosed with stage IV non-small cell lung cancer and meets with his oncologist to discuss the imaging findings and treatment options going forward. The oncologist informs the patient that his disease is terminal and that with existing treatments, he will likely live for another 6 months to 1 year. Near the end of the appointment, the oncologist ponders whether she should initiate a discussion about end-of-life issues. She hesitates because she does not want to demoralize him further and feels this can be addressed at future visits. What should she do?

Suggested Answer

Given this patient's disease and prognosis, national oncologic society guidelines recommend that his oncologist initiate a conversation about EOL care soon after the diagnosis of advanced cancer is made. It can take time for patients to process that their life is ending. Earlier discussions may give patients more opportunity to think about the type of EOL care that would best fit with their values and goals.

In this study, Mack and colleagues demonstrated that a large proportion of patients with stage IV lung or colon cancer do not participate in an EOL discussion until the last 30 days of life. Additionally, a majority of patients do not have this discussion until they are hospitalized. The study found that patients who did partake in EOL conversations before the last 30 days of life were significantly less likely to receive aggressive EOL medical care. This was also true for patients who had initial EOL conversation outside of the inpatient hospital setting.

Though aggressive EOL care may fit with the values and goals of some patients with advanced cancer, this is not the case for the majority. Earlier EOL discussions may help to ensure that patients with advanced caner have the opportunity to express their values and receive EOL care that reflects their preferences. Thus the physician should initiate an EOLd at this point in the patient's care.

References

1. Mack JW, Cronin A, Keating NL, et al. Associations between end-of-life discussion characteristics and care received near death: a prospective cohort study. *J Clin Oncol.* 2012 Dec 10;30(35):4387–4395.

2. Ayanian JZ, Chrischilles EA, Fletcher RH, et al. Understanding cancer treatment and outcomes: the Cancer Care Outcomes Research and Surveillance Consortium. *J Clin Oncol.* 2004 Dec 15;22(24):2992–2996.

3. Wright, AA, Zhang B, Ray A, et al. Associations between end-of-life discussions, patient mental health, medical care near death, and caregiver bereavement adjustment. *JAMA.* 2008 Oct 8;300(14):1665–1673.

4. Mack JW, Weeks JC, Wright AA, et al. End-of-life discussions, goal attainment, and distress at the end of life: predictors and outcomes of receipt of care consistent with preferences. *J Clin Oncol.* 2010 Mar 1;28(7):1203–1208.

5. National Comprehensive Cancer Network. Practice guidelines in oncology: Palliative care. Retrieved from http://www.nccn.org/professionals/physician_gls/f_guidelines.asp

6. Peppercorn JM, Smith TJ, Helft PR, et al. American Society of Clinical Oncology statement: Toward individualized care for patients with advanced cancer. *J Clin Oncol.* 2011 Feb 20;29(6):755–760.

7. Weeks JC, Catalano PJ, Cronin A, et al. Patients' expectations about effects of chemotherapy for advanced cancer. *N Engl J Med.* 2012 Oct 25;367(17):1616–1625.

8. Wright AA, Keating NL, Ayanian JZ, et al. Family perspectives on aggressive cancer care near the end of life. *JAMA.* 2016 Jan 19;315(3):284–292.

38

A Communication Intervention in the Intensive Care Unit

LORI OLSON AND CHRISTIAN T. SINCLAIR

[The] main goals [of end-of-life family conferences are] to improve communication between ICU staff and family members and to assist families when difficult decisions need to be made.

—LAUTRETTE ET AL.[1]

Research Question: Does a structured end-of-life family conference and written bereavement resources reduce the presence and severity of posttraumatic stress disorder (PTSD), anxiety, and depression in family members after the death of a patient in the intensive care unit (ICU)?

Funding: Assistance Publique-Hôpitaux de Paris, French Society for Critical Care Medicine.

Year Study Began: 2005.

Year Study Published: 2007.

Study Location: 22 ICUs in France.

Who Was Studied: Family members of critically ill patients believed to be imminently dying.

Who Was Excluded: Patients less than 18 years of age, family members with insufficient French literacy to conduct a telephone interview.

How Many Patients: 126.

Study Overview: This is an unblinded randomized controlled trial in which surrogates at each ICU were assigned to an intervention (n = 63) or control group (n = 63).

Patients in both groups received usual critical care, including 3 early formal family informational meetings within the first 5 days of the ICU stay as well as an end-of-life conference to inform family members of their loved ones' imminent death (Figure 38.1).

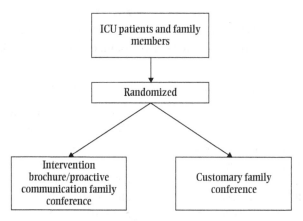

Figure 38.1 Summary of study design.

Study Intervention: For the intervention group, investigators led the structured end-of-life family conference utilizing the VALUE mnemonic with 5 main goals: **v**alue and appreciate what family members said; **a**cknowledge family members' emotions; **l**isten; ask questions to **u**nderstand who the patient was as a person; and **e**licit questions from family members. At the conclusion of the conference, surrogates were given a 15-page leaflet that described end-of-life care, possible grief reactions after a death, and resources regarding communication with loved ones about end of life and bereavement.

Patients in the control group received usual critical care. The end-of-life family conference discussing imminent death was conducted in the normal manner at each site. No brochure on bereavement was given to the surrogates.

Follow-up: A telephone interview was conducted 90 days after the patient's death with the surrogate; 86% of family members completed the follow-up interview.

Endpoints:

Primary outcome:
- Impact Event Scale (IES), which assesses PTSD burden at 3 months.[2]

Secondary outcome:
- Hospital Anxiety and Depression Scale (HADS), which evaluates presence and severity of anxiety and depression at 3 months.[3]

RESULTS

- At 3 months after the patient's death, surrogates in the intervention group had lower IES scores and lower HADS scores than those in the control group. Fewer surrogates in the intervention group had clinically significant symptoms of anxiety, depression, or PTSD (Table 38.1).

Table 38.1. SUMMARY OF STUDY'S KEY FINDINGS

	Control Group	Intervention Group	P Value
Conference and Clinical Care Variables			
Family expressed patient wishes	54%	70%	0.04
Nurse present	60%	81%	0.03
Median duration of conference (mins) (IQR)	20 (15–30)	30 (19–45)	<0.001
Median total time family spoke (mins) (IQR)	5 (5–10)	13.5 (8–20)	<0.001
Family-reported expression of emotions	75%	95%	0.03
Mechanical ventilation withdrawn?	14%	27%	0.03
Vasopressors withdrawn?	30%	51%	0.01
Caregiver Outcomes at 90 Days			
Median Impact Event Scale (IQR)[a]	39 (25–48)	27 (18–42)	0.02
Median HADS score (IQR)[b]	17 (11–25)	11 (8–18)	0.004
Anxiety symptoms in family	67%	45%	0.02
Depression symptoms in family	56%	29%	0.003

NOTE: IQR = Interquartile range; HADS = Hospital Anxiety and Depression Scale.

[a] 0 = no posttraumatic stress disorder–related symptoms; maximum score is 75.
[b] 0 = no distress; maximum score is 21.

- Surrogates more frequently expressed the patient's wishes and felt able to express their emotions to the critical care team in the structured end-of-life family conference. The conference in the intervention group

typically lasted 10 minutes longer with surrogates talking more than those in the control group.
- Patients in the intervention group received fewer nonbeneficial treatments (mechanical ventilation, vasopressors).

Criticisms and Limitations:

- The study was not designed to evaluate how much impact each variable in the intervention had in the outcome of the study. Specifically, no questions were asked regarding the value of the bereavement brochure.
- The outcomes measured were a snapshot 3 months after the patient's death and may not reflect family feelings at other time points, including prior to the patient's death.

Other Relevant Studies and Information:

- Patients and families identify quality ICU-palliative care as timely, concise, and compassionate communication by providers; plans of care selected based on patients' wishes; patient care focused on maintaining comfort and dignity; and interdisciplinary support for patients and families including bereavement for loved ones in the event of the death of a patient.[4]
- A previous study revealed that almost a third of the time a VALUE-based objective was not met during end-of-life family conferences.[5]
- The research network that performed this study also created and validated a tool assessing the experience of relatives of patients who die in the ICU. Utilizing this tool as a primary outcome in future studies will better evaluate whether future interventions impact the well-being of surrogates.[7]
- The results of this study support the recommendations by the American College of Critical Care Medicine for patient- and family-centered care alongside bereavement support for family members of patients expected to die in the ICU.[6]

Summary and Implications: In surrogates of patients dying in the ICU, an end-of-life family conference conducted according to VALUE-based guidelines along with written bereavement education reduced symptoms of PTSD, anxiety, and depression at 90 days after the death. This study highlights the role of family conference and how the skillful use of communication techniques can have a meaningful impact on patient and caregiver outcomes.

CLINICAL CASE: HOW DO WE BEST SUPPORT SERIOUSLLY ILL PATIENTS AND THEIR FAMILIES IN THE ICU?

Case History

In the monthly ICU meeting, the nurse supervisor notes that several deaths had really impacted the nurses, doctors, and social workers. Several of these patients had been cared for in the ICU by the same staff over long periods. When decisions were made to change goals to comfort, the nurses and social workers felt they had not been included in the discussions despite knowing the patient and family very well—so well, in fact, that some families contacted staff after the patient died in the ICU to express reservations about the decisions they made along with signs of depression and anxiety. The ICU staff are wondering if there is a better way to handle these situations in the future.

Suggested Answer

The randomized control trial by Lautrette et al. helps us understand how to impact ICU care of seriously ill patients at the system level. Having a few clinicians who are "better" at talking to patients and families about challenging medical decision-making still puts many families at risk of longer term mental health morbidity after a stressful ICU stay with a patient. Palliative care consult teams are increasingly more available in the ICU, but they may not be able to see all seriously ill patients.

Helping ICU teams build proactive communication skills helps families and patients express wishes, values, and goals so that care can be more concordant. Taking an interprofessional approach can help provide insights from various viewpoints and meet unique needs not matched by a biomedical model. Systematic availability of bereavement resources in the areas of the hospital with the highest risk of mortality and subsequent family psychological morbidity can support people during a vulnerable and emotional time.

The ICU nurse supervisor should coordinate with the ICU and palliative care teams to ensure adequate access in the ICU and identify resources for communication training and bereavement services in the ICU.

References

1. Lautrette A, Darmon M, Megarbane B, et al. A communication strategy and brochure for relatives of patients dying in the ICU. *N Engl J Med.* 2007 Feb 1;356(5):469–478.

2. Sundin EC, Horowitz MJ. Horowitz's Impact of Event Scale: evaluation of 20 years of use. *Psychosom Med.* 2003;65:870–876.

3. Zigmond AS, Snaith RP. The Hospital Anxiety and Depression Scale. *Acta Psychiatr Scand.* 1983;67:361–370.

4. Nelson JE, Puntillo KA, Pronovost PJ, et al. In their own words: patients and families define high-quality palliative care in the intensive care unit. *Crit Care Med.* 2010;38(3):808–818.

5. Curtis JR, Engelberg RA, Wenrich MD, et al. Missed opportunities during family conferences about end-of-life care in the intensive care unit. *Am J Respir Crit Care Med.* 2005 Apr;171:844–849.

6. Truog RD, Campbell ML, Curtis JR, et al. Recommendations for end-of-life care in the intensive care unit: a consensus statement by the American College of Critical Care Medicine. *Crit Care Med.* 2008;36:953–963.

7. Kentish-Barnes, N., Seegers, V., Legriel, S. et al. CAESAR: a new tool to assess relatives' experience of dying and death in the ICU. *Intensive Care Med.* 2016 June;42:95–1002.

Clinical Signs of Impending Death in Cancer Patients

MASANORI MORI

The physical signs reported here may pave the way toward the development and validation of a bedside diagnostic tool for impending death.
—HUI ET AL.[1]

Research Question: How often and when do patients with advanced cancer develop physical signs of impending death, and what is their diagnostic accuracy?

Funding: National Institutes of Health (CA 016672).

Year Study Began: 2010.

Year Study Published: 2015.

Study Location: Acute Palliative Care Units (APCUs) at the MD Anderson Cancer Center in the United States and Barretos Cancer Hospital in Brazil.

Who Was Studied: Advanced cancer patients admitted to the APCUs.

Who Was Excluded: None.

How Many Patients: 357.

Study Overview: The Investigating the Process of Dying Study was a prospective, longitudinal observational study to determine the frequency and onset of clinical signs associated with impending death and to determine their diagnostic performance (i.e., sensitivity, specificity, and negative and positive likelihood ratios) for impending death in 3 days. Nurses documented a total of 62 clinical signs every 12 hours. The former article reported 10 major clinical signs[2] and the latter 52 signs (Figure 39.1).[1]

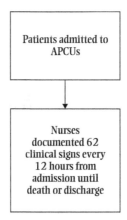

Figure 39.1 Summary of study design.

Study Intervention: Not applicable

Follow-up: Until death or discharge.

Endpoints: Prevalence of each studied sign in last 3 days of life, time from onset of each sign to death (days), and diagnostic utility of each sign.

RESULTS

- In total, 203 of 357 patients died in the APCU. The median duration of the APCU admission was 6 days (Table 39.1).
- The first article showed 3 "early signs" of impending death (i.e., Palliative Performance Scale (PPS) < 20%, Richmond Agitation

Table 39.1. Frequencies, Onsets Odds Ratios, Sensitivities, Specificities, and Negative and Positive LRs for Physical Signs in 3 Days

	Prevalence of Signs in Last 3 Days of Life, N (%)	Time From Onset to Death (Days), Median	Sens	Spec	LR–	LR+
PPS ≤20	169 (93%)	4	64	81.3	0.44	3.5
RASS –2 or lower	159 (90%)	7	50.5	89.3	0.6	4.9
Dysphagia of liquids	100 (90%)	7	40.9	78.8	0.75	1.9
Urine output over last 12 hours <100 mL	48 (72%)	1.5	24.2	98.2	0.77	15.2
Death rattle	110 (66%)	1.5	22.4	97.1	0.8	9
Apnea periods	71 (46%)	1.5	17.6	95.3	0.86	4.5
Respiration with mandibular movement	92 (56%)	1.5	22	97.5	0.8	10
Peripheral cyanosis	99 (59%)	3	26.7	94.9	0.77	5.7
Cheyne-Stokes breathing	61 (41%)	2	14.1	98.5	0.9	12.4
Pulselessness of radial artery	57 (38%)	1	11.3	99.3	0.89	15.6
Decreased response to verbal stimuli	118 (69%)	2.0	30	96	0.73	8.3
Decreased response to visual stimuli	121 (70%)	3.0	31.9	94.9	0.72	6.7
Nonreactive pupils	53 (38%)	2.0	15.3	99	0.86	16.7
Drooping of nasolabial fold	137 (78%)	2.5	33.7	95.5	0.69	8.3
Hyperextension of neck	73 (46%)	2.5	21.2	96.7	0.82	7.3
Inability to close eyelids	93 (57%)	1.5	21.4	97.9	0.8	13.6
Grunting of vocal cords	86 (54%)	1.5	19.5	97.9	0.82	11.8
Upper gastrointestinal bleed	6 (5%)	5.5	2.9	99.7	0.97	10.3

NOTE: LR = likelihood ratio; Sens. = sensitivity; Spec. = specificity; LR– = negative likelihood ratio; LR+ = positive likelihood ratio; PPS = Palliative Performance Scale; RASS = Richmond Agitation Sedation Scale.

Sedation Scale (RASS) –2 or lower, and dysphagia of liquids) and 7 "late signs" (i.e., urine output over last 12 hours < 100 mL, death rattle, apnea periods, respiration with mandibular movement, peripheral cyanosis, Cheyne-Stokes breathing, and pulselessness of radial artery).[2] While early signs had a high prevalence over the last 3 days of life (90%–93%), and a median onset ranging from 4 to 7 days prior to death, their diagnostic performance was not high with positive likelihood ratios (LRs) less than 5 for impending death in 3 days.

- In contrast, late signs had a lower frequency (38%–72%) and a median onset of 3 days or less before death; however, their diagnostic performance was high with high specificity (>95%) and high positive LR (4.5–15.6).
- The second article revealed that a total of 7 neurological signs (i.e., nonreactive pupils, decreased response to verbal stimuli, decreased response to visual stimuli, inability to close eyelids, drooping of the nasolabial fold, hyperextension of the neck, and grunting of the vocal cord) had increasing frequency over the last 3 days of life and had a late median onset within the last 3 days of life. They had high specificity (>95%) and a high positive LR (6.7–16.7) associated with death within 3 days (Table 39.1).[1] Upper gastrointestinal bleeding also had high specificity and positive LR, though its frequency was only 5%.
- The multivariate analysis revealed that a decreased response to verbal stimuli (odds ratio, 6.61; 95% confidence interval 2.49–23.17; P = 0.0004) and drooping of the nasolabial fold (odds ratio, 6.51; 95% confidence interval 2.67–20.07; P = 0.0001) were significantly associated with death within 3 days.[1]

Criticisms and Limitations:

- This study included only cancer patients admitted to APCUs, who often have severe distress. Caution should be taken when these findings are applied in other settings.
- The interrater reliability of these clinical signs was not formally confirmed.
- The sample size was relatively small for a large number of clinical signs, and the signs were collected every 12 hours, which limited the resolution of data.
- These findings should be considered preliminary, and further studies are warranted to validate them prospectively.

Other Relevant Studies and Information:

- A previous landmark study showed that the mean (median) time from the onset of death rattle, respiration with mandibular movement (RMM), cyanosis on extremities, and pulselessness on the radial artery to death was 57 (23) hours, 7.6 (2.5) hours, 5.1 (1.0) hours, and 2.6 (1.0) hours, respectively.[3]
- An international Delphi revealed that changes in "breathing," "general deterioration," "consciousness/cognition," "skin," "intake of fluid, food, others," "emotional state" and "non-observations/expressed opinions/ other" were considered highly predictive of impending death.[4]
- The Investigating the Process of Dying Study also demonstrated that (1) the proportion of patients able to communicate decreased from 80% to 39% over the last 7 days of life;[5] (2) anorexia, drowsiness, fatigue, poor well-being, and dyspnea worsened significantly as death approached, while depression decreased over time; and (3) blood pressure and oxygen saturation decreased significantly in the final 3 days of life.[6]
- The study also produced a diagnostic model for impending death based on two variables (PPS and drooping of nasolabial folds) and had four terminal leaves in a decision tree: PPS score ≤ 20% and drooping of nasolabial folds present, PPS score ≤ 20% and drooping of nasolabial folds absent, PPS score of 30% to 60%, and PPS score ≥ 70%. The 3-day mortality rates were 94%, 42%, 16%, and 3%, respectively (accuracy, 81%).[7]
- The Objective Palliative Prognostic Score was developed to estimate 7-day survival. If any 3 of the 6 objective predictors (heart rate >120/ min, white blood cells >11,000/mm^3, platelets <130,000/mm^3, serum creatinine level >1.3 mg/dL, serum potassium level >5 mg/dL, and no history of chemotherapy) were reached, death within 7 days was predicted with 68.8% sensitivity, 86.0% specificity, 55.9% positive predictive value, and 91.4% negative predictive value.[8]

Summary and Implications: This is the first study to systematically characterize the frequency, onset, and diagnostic performance of 62 clinical signs of impending death in patients with advanced cancer admitted to APCUs. In particular, 7 "late signs," in conjunction with 7 neurological signs (i.e., decreased response to verbal stimuli, decreased response to visual stimuli, nonreactive pupils, drooping of nasolabial fold, hyperextension of neck, inability to close eyelids, grunting of vocal cords) and upper gastrointestinal bleeding, have high positive LRs for impending death within 3 days. Upon further validation, these signs may assist clinicians in predicting impending death.

CLINICAL CASE: WHEN SHOULD FAMILIES GATHER AND STAY WITH THE PATIENT?

Case History

A 60-year-old man with metastatic pancreatic cancer has progressed through 3 lines of chemotherapies and has no further treatment options. His general condition has deteriorated rapidly over the past few weeks. Currently his performance status is 4, and he has decreasing oral intake with dysphagia of liquids. He has had worsening upper abdominal pain over the past 3 days and is admitted to the APCU for symptom management. In the evening of the day of admission, his pain is relieved with opioid titration. However, he now develops RMM. Both the patient and his wife are aware of his poor prognosis. Their grown-up children live far away from the area but always wanted to take days off from work to stay with their father should his death be imminent. His wife asks you if she should call their children.

Suggested Answer

This patient has already shown early signs (PPS ≤20% and dysphagia of liquids) prior to the admission, indicating that he is deteriorating. A majority of patients present with early signs in the last days of life, but because of their lower specificity, the presence of early signs alone cannot inform us that death is imminent.

However, he developed RMM soon after the admission. This is one of the late signs and has very high specificity (97.5%) and high positive LR (10) of impending death. Assuming that the pretest probability for dying within 3 days of admission to this APCU is 30%, the presence of RMM results in a posttest probability of greater than 80% of death within the next 3 days. Given this information, in conjunction with the evidence that the median time from the onset of RMM to death is 1.5 days, the patient's wife should be informed that his death is imminent and be advised that she call their children immediately.

References

1. Hui D, Dos Santos R, Chisholm G, Bansal S, Souza Crovador C, Bruera E. Bedside clinical signs associated with impending death in patients with advanced cancer: preliminary findings of a prospective, longitudinal cohort study. *Cancer.* 2015 Mar 15;121(6):960–967.
2. Hui D, dos Santos R, Chisholm G, et al. Clinical signs of impending death in cancer patients. *Oncologist.* 2014 Jun;19(6):681–687.

3. Morita T, Ichiki T, Tsunoda J, Inoue S, Chihara S. A prospective study on the dying process in terminally ill cancer patients. *Am J Hospice Palliat Care.* 1998 Jul-Aug;15(4):217–222.

4. Domeisen Benedetti F, Ostgathe C, Clark J, et al. International palliative care experts' view on phenomena indicating the last hours and days of life. *Support Care Cancer.* 2013 Jun;21(6):1509–1517.

5. Hui D, dos Santos R, Chisholm GB, Bruera E. Symptom expression in the last seven days of life among cancer patients admitted to acute palliative care units. *J Pain Symptom Manage.* 2015 Oct;50(4):488–494.

6. Bruera S, Chisholm G, Dos Santos R, Crovador C, Bruera E, Hui D. Variations in vital signs in the last days of life in patients with advanced cancer. *J Pain Symptom Manage.* 2014 Oct;48(4):510–517.

7. Hui D, Hess K, dos Santos R, Chisholm G, Bruera E. A diagnostic model for impending death in cancer patients: preliminary report. *Cancer.* 2015 Nov 1;121(21):3914–3921.

8. Chen YT, Ho CT, Hsu HS, et al. Objective palliative prognostic score among patients with advanced cancer. *J Pain Symptom Manage.* 2015 Apr;49(4):690–696.

Factors Considered Important at the End of Life

RAVI B. PARIKH AND OREOFE O. ODEJIDE

> The results of this survey suggest that for patients and families, physical care is expectedly crucial, but is only one component of total care.
> —STEINHAUSER ET AL.[1]

Research Question: What factors do patients, families, physicians, and other care providers consider important at the end of life?

Funding: Veterans Affairs (VA), Robert Wood Johnson Generalist Physician Faculty Scholars Award, and Soros Foundation Project on Death in America Faculty Scholars Program.

Year Study Began: 1999.

Year Study Published: 2000.

Study Location: VA medical centers across the United States.

Who Was Studied: VA patients with cancer, end-stage renal failure, congestive heart failure, or chronic obstructive pulmonary disease hospitalized in the year prior to study enrollment. Also included were family members of VA patients who died 6 to 12 months earlier, as well as physicians and other care providers (nurses, social workers, chaplains, and hospice volunteers) for patients at the end of life.

Who Was Excluded: Patients, bereaved family members, physicians, and other care providers who did not respond to the survey.

How Many Patients: 340 patients, 332 bereaved family members, 361 physicians, and 429 other care providers (97 nurses, 107 social workers, 120 chaplains, 105 hospice volunteers).

Study Overview: This was a cross-sectional, mailed national survey, stratified by participant type. Respondents were asked to rate the importance of 44 attributes at the end of life on a 5-point Likert scale (strongly disagree to strongly agree) and were also asked to rank 9 items in order of importance (Figure 40.1).

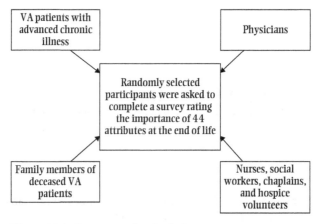

Figure 40.1 Summary of study design.

Study Intervention: Not applicable.

Follow-up: Not applicable.

Endpoints: Primary outcome: Importance of 44 attributes of quality at the end of life and ranking of 9 major attributes.

RESULTS

- Among 1,885 participants, 1,462 (78%) responded to the survey. Response rate by participant group was 77% among patients, 71%

among bereaved family members, 74% among physicians, and 88% among other care providers.

- 26 items were consistently rated as important by all four groups of participants (>70% agreed that attribute is important). These items involved pain and symptom management, preparation for death; achieving a sense of completion about one's life, decisions about treatment preferences; being treated as a whole person, and patients' relationships with health care professionals.
- 8 items were of strong importance to patients but were significantly less important to physicians, including being mentally aware and coming to peace with God (Table 40.1).

Table 40.1. SUMMARY OF STUDY'S KEY FINDINGS

Attribute	Participants Who Agreed That Attribute Is Important	
	Patients N = 340 (%)	Physicians N = 361 (%)
Be mentally aware	92	65
Be at peace with God	89	65
Not be a burden to family	89	58
Be able to help others	88	44
Pray	85	55
Have funeral arrangements planned	82	58
Not be a burden to society	81	44
Feel one's life is complete	80	68

- In adjusted multivariable models, physicians (odds ratio [OR] 0.1, 95% confidence interval [CI] 0.1–0.2) and other care providers (OR 0.08, 95% CI 0.04–0.14) were significantly less likely than patients to agree with the importance of using all available treatments regardless of the chance of recovery, while bereaved family members were equally as likely. Other care providers were more likely than patients to agree that dying at home is important (OR 1.7, 95% CI 1.1–2.0), whereas physicians and bereaved family members were not significantly different from patients. Physicians (OR 2.0, 95% CI 1.3–2.5), other care providers (OR 1.7, 95% CI 1.1–2.0), and bereaved family members (OR 1.7, 95% CI 1.1–2.7) were all more likely than patients to agree that talking about the meaning of death is important.
- When asked to rank 9 preselected attributes, all groups ranked freedom from pain as most important. Dying at home was ranked least important by all groups except other care providers, who ranked it second to last.

Criticisms and Limitations:

- The study population included VA patients and their family members, which may limit generalization to other settings.
- Individuals included in the other care provider group typically engage in patient care in diverse settings (i.e., nurses in disease-directed treatment settings to hospice volunteers focused on comfort care). Given the degree of heterogeneity, their perspectives on attributes of good end-of-life care may vary considerably within the group.

Other Relevant Studies and Information:

- It has been demonstrated that patients often receive overly intensive care at the end of life that may be inconsistent with their values.[2] Accordingly, several efforts have focused on developing frameworks for quality of end-of-life care. Initial work was based largely on medical experts' perspectives of end-of-life care.[3,4]
- Early work to characterize patients' views was conducted by Singer and colleagues through in-depth interviews.[5] Five domains of quality end-of-life care emerged: receiving adequate pain and symptom management, avoiding inappropriate prolongation of dying, achieving a sense of control, relieving burden, and strengthening relationships with loved ones.
- Steinhauser et al. further broadened the taxonomy for end-of-life care by gathering descriptions of what constitutes a good death from patients, families, and providers through 12 focus groups.[6] Six major components of a good death were identified, including pain and symptom management, decision-making, preparation for death, completion, contributing to others, and affirmation of the whole person. These findings formed the basis of the national survey discussed in this chapter.
- End-of-life frameworks such as the one developed from this survey and others[1,7] have been employed to develop instruments to assess quality of end-of-life care from the perspectives of patients and bereaved family members,[8,9] thus informing efforts for improvement.
- Given the broad variation in the definition of what constitutes a good death, it is critical for physicians to conduct timely discussions to elicit their patients' preferences regarding end-of-life care.

Summary and Implications: This cross-sectional survey study by Steinhauser and colleagues helps to define a "good death" from the perspectives of key stakeholders. All stakeholders identified pain and symptom management and strong relationships between patients and health professionals as very important. Preparation for the end of life was also consistently considered important, highlighting the need for honest and timely prognostic conversations. For patients but less so for physicians, being mentally aware and attention to spirituality were of strong importance. These findings highlight the need for physicians to meticulously elicit their patients' values regarding quality care and incorporate them into end-of-life decision-making and care.

CLINICAL CASE: WHAT END-OF-LIFE FACTORS ARE IMPORTANT TO A PATIENT?

Case History

A 60-year-old man with metastatic lung cancer whose disease is progressive with new bony metastases presents for an appointment with his oncologist. The oncologist attempts to elicit the patient's goals of care. While both agree that pain control is the most important treatment priority, the oncologist is surprised to hear from the patient, "I only want something to take the edge off the pain. I want to be awake for these last few weeks." How should the physician respond?

Suggested Answer

The physician in this case assumes that this patient with a poor prognosis is solely interested in the treatment of his pain, which is arguably the most important symptom consideration in patients with metastatic cancer. The landmark SUPPORT study showed that a substantial proportion of patients with serious illness such as cancer live with uncontrolled symptoms such as moderate to severe pain.[2]

Although freedom from pain was ranked as the most important attribute of a good death by patients and physicians in the study by Steinhauser and colleagues, there are additional key attributes that are important to patients relating to broader psychosocial and spiritual issues that are often not recognized by physicians. For example, being mentally aware was strongly important to patients in this study but not to physicians. In addition, the mean difference in the ranking of pain control and mental awareness by patients was much smaller compared to physicians, indicating that patients are less willing to sacrifice mental awareness for pain control. The patient in this case is expressing that his desire is not solely for pain control at the end of life but also for lucidity.

Other attributes that may be important to patients but less recognized by physicians include the desire not to be a burden to family or society, being at peace with God, and praying. Physicians and other care team members may also underestimate the extent to which patients and their family members consider use of all available treatments no matter the chance of recovery to be important.

The oncologist in this case should be aware of patients' varying expectations at the end of life and engage in a nonprescriptive discussion to determine the most patient-centered care plan going forward.

References

1. Steinhauser KE, Christakis NA, Clipp EC, McNeilly M, McIntyre L, Tulsky JA. Factors considered important at the end of life by patients, family, physicians, and other care providers. *JAMA*. 2000;284:2476–2482.
2. SUPPORT Principal Investigators. A controlled trial to improve care for seriously ill hospitalized patients. The Study to Understand Prognoses and Preferences for Outcomes and Risks of Treatments (SUPPORT). *JAMA*. 1995;274:1591–1598.
3. Lynn J. Measuring quality of care at the end of life: a statement of principles. *J Am Geriatr Soc*. 1997;45:526–527.
4. Emanuel EJ, Emanuel LL. The promise of a good death. *Lancet*. 1998;351(Suppl 2):SII21–SII29.
5. Singer PA, Martin DK, Kelner M. Quality end-of-life care: patients' perspectives. *JAMA*. 1999;281:163–168.
6. Steinhauser KE, Clipp EC, McNeilly M, Christakis NA, McIntyre LM, Tulsky JA. In search of a good death: observations of patients, families, and providers. *Ann Intern Med*. 2000;132:825–832.
7. Teno JM, Casey VA, Welch LC, Edgman-Levitan S. Patient-focused, family-centered end-of-life medical care: views of the guidelines and bereaved family members. *J Pain Symptom Manage*. 2001;22:738–751.
8. Steinhauser KE, Clipp EC, Bosworth HB, et al. Measuring quality of life at the end of life: validation of the QUAL-E. *Palliat Support Care*. 2004;2:3–14.
9. Steinhauser KE, Voils CI, Bosworth HB, Tulsky JA. Validation of a measure of family experience of patients with serious illness: the QUAL-E (Fam). *J Pain Symptom Manage*. 2014;48:1168–1181.

Quality End-of-Life Care

Patients' Perspectives

JESSE A. SOODALTER AND YAEL SCHENKER

[T]he purpose of this study was to identify and describe elements of quality end-of-life care as identified by those most affected: patients.

—SINGER ET AL.[1]

Research Question: What are the elements of quality end-of-life (EOL) care, as perceived by patients?

Funding: National Health Research and Development Program, Ottawa, Ontario; Medical Research Council of Canada; Physicians' Services Incorporated Foundation of Ontario.

Year Study Began: 1994.

Year Study Published: 1999.

Study Location: 6 adult hemodialysis units, a HIV clinic and a long-term care facility, all in Toronto, Canada.

Who Was Studied: Hemodialysis patients interviewed in a prior trial examining advance care planning preferences,[2] persons infected with HIV interviewed in a prior trial comparing preferences between a generic advance directive (AD) form and an HIV/AIDS-specific AD form,[3] and residents of a long-term care facility interviewed in a prior trial exploring preferences about control at the EOL.[4]

Who Was Excluded: Dialysis patients: age <18 years, unable to understand written English, incapable of completing an AD or likely to experience undue emotional distress from form completion, and those with <3 months on dialysis. HIV patients: age <16 years, non-English-fluent, incapable of completing an AD (as measured by Standardized Mini-Mental State Exam score <23) or likely to experience undue emotional distress from completing an AD form, resided outside metropolitan Toronto. Long-term care residents: age <65 years, incapable of understanding and answering questions in English, too physically or mentally ill to participate.

How Many Patients: 126: dialysis (n = 48), HIV (n = 40, randomly selected from 140 interviews), long-term care (n = 38).

Study Overview: This study explored patients' views on quality EOL care by performing content analysis on in-depth, open-ended interview data from three previous interview studies. These studies examined preferences regarding advance care planning (in dialysis patients and individuals with HIV/AIDS) and EOL control (in elderly long-term care residents). For the current study, respondents' views regarding quality EOL care were identified from the original interviews, coded by underlining and writing descriptive notes in the margins, and then given labels describing specific EOL care issues. The labeled issues were compared both within and between interviews and grouped into overarching domains, whereupon the investigators recoded the transcripts by reading them again and assigning relevant passages to the newly-identified domains (Figure 41.1).

Study Intervention: Not applicable.

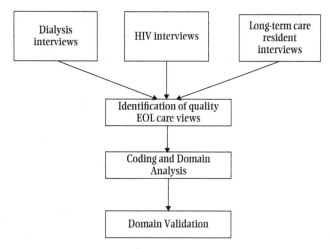

Figure 41.1 Summary of study design.

Follow-up: Not applicable.

Endpoints: Patient-expressed domains of quality EOL care.

RESULTS

- Five domains of quality EOL care were identified:
  - Receiving adequate pain and symptom management
  - Avoiding inappropriate prolongation of dying
  - Achieving a sense of control
  - Relieving burden [on loved ones]
  - Strengthening relationships with loved ones
- Compared with three other recently published taxonomies of quality EOL care by expert groups, the authors noted the patient-derived taxonomy to be both simpler and more specific, less focused on psychometrically driven concepts like "quality of life" and processes of care, and more focused on outcomes (Table 41.1).

Table 41.1. DOMAINS OF QUALITY EOL CARE BY PARTICIPANT GROUP

Domain	Dialysis Participants n (%)	HIV/AIDS Participants n (%)	Long-Term Care Participants n (%)	Total N (%)
Receiving adequate pain and symptom management	3 (6)	10 (25)	15 (40)	28 (22)
Avoiding inappropriate prolongation of dying	23 (48)	29 (73)	25 (66)	77 (61)
Achieving a sense of control	9 (19)	21 (53)	18 (47)	48 (38)
Relieving burden	14 (29)	21 (53)	13 (34)	48 (38)
Strengthening relationships with loved ones	16 (33)	21 (53)	12 (32)	49 (39)

NOTE: EOL = end-of-life.

Criticisms and Limitations:

- This was a secondary analysis of interviews that were not designed to elicit participants' EOL care views. Topics such as spirituality or financial concerns that figure prominently in other taxonomies are absent in this model.
- The race/ethnicity of the sample was predominantly white (81%), with African Americans representing 6% and Hispanics and Asians each 2% of respondents. This likely limits the study's generalizability, particularly since ethnicity and culture are known to influence EOL care perceptions.

Other Relevant Studies and Information:

- Steinhauser et al. published a large (N = 1,462) national survey of patients, family, physicians, and care providers assessing the importance of 44 attributes of EOL care and classifying the results by category and degree of agreement among subgroups.[5] This study found that while "freedom from pain" ranked first among nine preselected attributes for all groups, among patients and family members this item ranked nearly identically with being "at peace with God."
- A large (N = 600) Canadian study of seriously ill patients and their family members found that patients most frequently rated as "extremely important" the following elements of EOL care:[6]

- "To have trust and confidence in the doctors looking after you"
- "Not to be kept alive on life support when there is little hope for a meaningful recovery"
- "That information about your disease be communicated to you by your doctor in an honest manner"
- "To complete things and prepare for life's end—life review, resolving conflicts, saying goodbye"

Summary and Implications: This study established the centrality of patients' views in determining the key aspects of quality EOL care and highlighted the importance of assessing these views in a variety of different populations. Patients identified the following five domains to be their top priorities at the end of life: receiving adequate pain and symptom management, avoiding inappropriate prolongation of dying, achieving a sense of control, relieving burden, and strengthening relationships with loved ones.

CLINICAL CASE: WHAT DOES QUALITY EOL CARE LOOK LIKE FOR MY PATIENT?

Case History

Mrs. W is an 85-year-old African American woman with end-stage congestive heart failure, newly enrolled in hospice. She lives in a ground-floor apartment attached to the house of her daughter, the daughter's husband, and two young sons. The patient has no pain but becomes short of breath with minimal exertion, including some activities of daily living like bathing. Her daughter comes in to check on her and bring over meals at least once a day, but Mrs. W worries that these duties are an imposition on her daughter's busy life. She regrets the loss of her independence and also wishes she were in closer touch with her son, who lives in another state and seldom visits.

What are the most important aspects of Mrs. W's care in her last months of life?

Suggested Answer

The Singer et al. study highlights several aspects of care that may be important to this patient: symptom management, a sense of control, fear of burdening loved ones, and strengthening relationships. Several of these aspects can be addressed by team-based hospice care, including symptom medication, assistance with home care needs, and psychosocial support to address adjustment to illness and family breakdown.

Subsequent research demonstrates, however, that the specifics of desired EOL care are highly variable across individuals and populations, and it is possible that Mrs. W has concerns that are not evident from her history alone, such as spirituality or finances. Thus her hospice team may wish to engage with Mrs. W in exploring her own priorities for EOL care, using the Singer et al. domains or another evidence-based taxonomy as a basis for discussion.

References

1. Singer PA, Martin DK, Kelner M. Quality end-of-life care: patients' perspectives. *JAMA*. 1999;281(2):163–168.
2. Singer PA, Martin DK, Lavery JV, Thiel EC, Kelner M, Mendelssohn DC. Reconceptualizing advance care planning from the patient's perspective. *Arch Intern Med*. 1998;158(8):879–884.
3. Martin DK, Thiel EC, Singer PA. A new model of advance care planning: observations from people with hiv. *Arch Intern Med*. 1999;159(1):86–92.
4. Kelner M. Activists and delegators: Elderly patients' preferences about control at the end of life. *Social Sci Med*. 1995;41(4):537–545.
5. Steinhauser KE, Christakis NA, Clipp EC, McNeilly M, McIntyre L, Tulsky JA. Factors considered important at the end of life by patients, family, physicians, and other care providers. *JAMA*. 2000;284(19):2476–2482.
6. Heyland DK, Dodek P, Rocker G, et al. What matters most in end-of-life care: perceptions of seriously ill patients and their family members. *CMAJ*. 2006;174(5):627–633.

42

Family Perspectives on Aggressive End-of-Life Care

RAVI B. PARIKH AND OREOFE ODEJIDE

These findings are supportive of advance care planning consistent with the preferences of patients.

—WRIGHT ET AL.[1]

Research Question: How does aggressive end-of-life care for patients with cancer influence bereaved family members' perceptions of quality of end-of-life care and patients' receipt of goal-concordant care?

Funding: National Cancer Institute.

Year Study Began: 2003.

Year Study Published: 2016.

Study Location: 5 regions (northern California, Los Angeles County, North Carolina, Iowa, and Alabama) and 5 integrated health systems.

Who Was Studied: Medicare patients with advanced lung or colorectal cancer enrolled in the Cancer Care Outcomes Research and Surveillance (CanCORS) study aged 65 years or older, who died by the end of 2011, as well as their bereaved family members.

Who Was Excluded: Patients for whom there was no after-death interview from a family member, patients not continuously enrolled in Medicare Parts A and B fee-for-service as of 3 months before death, and patients for whom family members did not rate the quality of end-of-life care.

How Many Patients: 1,146 patients and family members.

Study Overview: Bereaved family members were asked to rate the quality of end-of-life care their loved one received and to assess whether the medical care received in the last month of life and location of death were congruent with the patient's wishes (Figure 42.1).

Study Intervention: Not applicable.

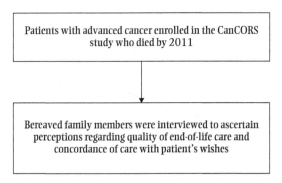

Figure 42.1 Summary of study design.

Follow-up: Not applicable.

Endpoints: Primary outcome: Family member-reported quality rating of end-of-life care, categorized into "excellent" versus other ("very good," "good," "fair," or "poor"). Secondary outcomes: Family member reports of patient goal attainment (i.e., extent to which end-of-life care was congruent with wishes and whether death occurred in preferred location).

RESULTS

- Among 1,146 cancer decedents, 51.3% of bereaved family members reported that quality of end-of-life care was excellent, 27.8% reported it to be very good, and 20.9% reported it to be good, fair, or poor.

- Family members reported that end-of-life wishes were followed a "great deal" in 81.1% of patients and "somewhat" or "not at all" in 18.9% of patients. Death occurred in patients' preferred location for 56.7% of those with a known preferred place of death.
- Patients who preferred life-prolonging therapies over symptom-directed care were significantly more likely to receive chemotherapy within 2 weeks of death and more likely to receive 3 or fewer days of hospice care. They were also more likely to have at least 2 hospital admissions in the last month of life and to die in the hospital.
- Family members rated end-of-life care as excellent more often for patients who received hospice care for longer than 3 days compared to those who did not (adjusted difference 16.5%; Table 42.1).

Table 42.1. SUMMARY OF STUDY'S KEY FINDINGS

Type of Aggressive End-of-Life Care	Family Member Reported Excellent End-of-Life Care (Total N = 1,146)		Family Member Reported that Death Occurred in Preferred Place (Total N = 774)	
	Adjusted %	P	Adjusted %	P
Intensive care unit admission during last month of life		0.04		<0.001
No	52.5		59.4	
Yes	43.1		36.6	
≥2 Hospitalizations during last month of life		0.17		0.27
No	51.8		57.1	
Yes	43.3		48.3	
≥2 Emergency department visits during last month of life		0.79		0.68
No	51.4		56.8	
Yes	49.9		54.1	
Chemotherapy ≤2 weeks before death		0.68		0.03
No	51.5		57.5	
Yes	48.9		39.8	
No hospice or ≤3 days before death		<0.001		<0.001
No	59.3		74.0	
Yes	42.8		39.6	
Death occurred in hospital		<0.001		<0.001
No	58.0		77.9	
Yes	41.0		27.4	

- Conversely, family members were less likely to report excellent end-of-life care for patients who had an intensive care unit (ICU) admission within 30 days of death or died in the hospital (Table 42.1).
- With respect to receipt of goal-concordant care, family members of patients who received 3 or fewer days of hospice care were less likely to report that their loved one's end-of-life wishes were followed. Aggressive end-of-life care (i.e., hospice care for 3 days or less, receipt of chemotherapy within 2 weeks of death, ICU admission, and death in the hospital) was associated with significantly lower likelihood of family member report that patient died in his or her preferred location (Table 42.1).

Criticisms and Limitations:

- The study population was restricted to Medicare enrollees, which may limit generalizability of the findings to younger, commercially insured, or uninsured individuals.
- One of the key outcomes for this study was overall perception, which was based on a single question ("Overall, how would you rate the care received [at the last place where care was provided]?) This has not been well validated and may not fully assess the multiple dimensional aspects of end-of-life care.
- Interviews of bereaved family members regarding their loved one's end-of-life care occurred at varying time points after death, which may introduce recall bias.

Other Relevant Studies and Information:

- Multiple studies have demonstrated that patients with advanced cancer are receiving increasingly aggressive care—such as chemotherapy, ICU admission, and terminal hospitalization—near the end of life.[2-4] In addition, although hospice use has increased, there has also been a concurrent rise in late hospice admissions (≤3 days before death).[2]
- This rising trend in aggressive cancer care at the end of life persists despite accruing data demonstrating that aggressive cancer care and absent or late hospice use are associated with worse patient quality of life and bereavement adjustment for caregivers.[5,6]
- Given the literature regarding the negative effects of overly aggressive medical care at the end of life, the American Society of Clinical Oncology has endorsed measures such as receipt of chemotherapy

within the last 2 weeks of life, repeated hospitalizations, emergency department visits, or ICU admission within the last month of life, and late or absent hospice admissions, as indicators of low-quality end-of-life care.[7]

- This study by Wright and colleagues lends additional credence to end-of-life quality measures by demonstrating that less aggressive end-of-life care significantly improves family members' perceptions of patient goal attainment.[1]

Summary and Implications: This large study of Medicare patients who died of lung or colorectal cancer demonstrates that measures such as earlier hospice enrollment and avoidance of ICU admissions and hospital deaths are associated with more positive family member perceptions of end-of-life care. These findings support efforts to encourage timely, high-quality goals of care discussions.

CLINICAL CASE: HOW DOES AGGRESSIVE END-OF-LIFE CARE IMPACT QUALITY OF CARE?

Case History

A 70-year-old man with stage IV lung cancer presents with his wife to his oncologist's office after a recent hospitalization for postobstructive pneumonia. He has been hospitalized twice in the past 3 months, one of which included a brief ICU admission, and his exercise tolerance has decreased significantly over the past 3 weeks. "We are sick of going back and forth to the hospital," the wife says, to the agreement of her husband.

How should the oncologist address the concern of the patient and his wife?

Suggested Answer

The patient in this scenario is experiencing repeated hospital admissions, and both he and his wife are voicing their distress with the multiple hospitalizations. The patient is near the end of life, and he is at risk of receiving increasingly aggressive care, which as demonstrated by Wright and colleagues is associated with poor ratings of quality of end-of-life care by family members. The concern expressed by the patient and his wife likely indicates a preference for less aggressive medical care.

As advocated by Wright and colleagues, advance care planning to elicit the patient's preferences are in order. Indeed, this visit and the concern raised by the patient and his wife provide an opportunity for the oncologist to more thoroughly explore the patient's treatment preferences. The oncologist should

attempt to elicit the patient's goals, values, and preferences regarding hospitalizations, location of death, as quality of end-of-life care is sensitive to these
preferences. Additionally, this would be an appropriate time to discuss hospice
care, given the limited life expectancy of this patient and the positive association of hospice with quality of end-of-life care. Eliciting the patient's preferences will help the oncologist provide care that is closely aligned with the
patient's wishes and may improve the wife's perception of the quality of care
provided.

References

1. Wright AA, Keating NL, Ayanian JZ, et al. Family perspectives on aggressive cancer
   care near the end of life. *JAMA*. 2016;315:284–292.
2. Earle CC, Landrum MB, Souza JM, Neville BA, Weeks JC, Ayanian JZ.
   Aggressiveness of cancer care near the end of life: Is it a quality-of-care issue? *J Clin
   Oncol*. 2008;26:3860–3866.
3. Ho TH, Barbera L, Saskin R, Lu H, Neville BA, Earle CC. Trends in the aggressiveness of end-of-life cancer care in the universal health care system of Ontario, Canada.
   J Clin Oncol. 2011;29:1587–1591.
4. Wright AA, Hatfield LA, Earle CC, Keating NL. End-of-life care for older patients
   with ovarian cancer is intensive despite high rates of hospice use. *J Clin Oncol*.
   2014;32:3534–3539.
5. Wright AA, Zhang B, Ray A, et al. Associations between end-of-life discussions,
   patient mental health, medical care near death, and caregiver bereavement adjustment. *JAMA*. 2008;300:1665–1673.
6. Kris AE, Cherlin EJ, Prigerson H, et al. Length of hospice enrollment and subsequent
   depression in family caregivers: 13-month follow-up study. *Am J Geratr Psychiatr*.
   2006;14:264–269.
7. Campion FX, Larson LR, Kadlubek PJ, Earle CC, Neuss MN. Advancing performance measurement in oncology: quality oncology practice initiative participation
   and quality outcomes. *J Oncol Pract*. 2011;7:31s–35s.

43

Family Perspectives on End-of-Life Care at the Last Place of Care

ESMÉ FINLAY AND ERIN FITZGERALD

> Bereaved family members of patients with home hospice services . . . reported higher satisfaction, fewer concerns with care, and fewer unmet needs.
> —TENO ET AL.[1]

Research Question: Are patient- and family-centered end-of-life outcomes different for patients dying at home versus in institutional settings?

Funding: Robert Wood Johnson Foundation (Grant 037188).

Year Study Began: 2000.

Year Study Published: 2004.

Study Location: United States.

Who Was Studied: Decedents who died in the United States, via telephone interviews with informants listed on patients' death certificates.

Who Was Excluded: Decedents <18 years old; decedents who died of trauma.

How Many Patients: 1,578 informant interviews were completed based on a sample of 3,275 decedents identified by death certificates.

Study Overview: This study is a mortality follow-back survey involving telephone interviews with family/informants of decedents who died in 2000. The authors used a 2-stage probability sample to identify a sample of patient deaths in 22 states. Bereaved informants were asked about the quality of patients' dying experience and the last place of care (Figure 43.1).

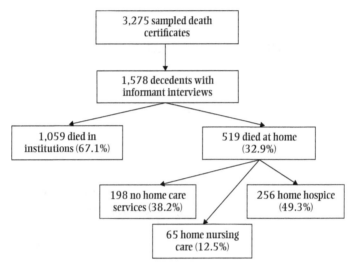

Figure 43.1 Summary of study design.

Study Intervention: Bereaved informants of deceased patients, identified by information on death certificates, completed telephone interviews about care received at the location where patients last spent 48 or more hours

Follow-up: Not applicable.

Endpoints: Outcome measures include whether health care providers met the following five patient- or family-oriented end-of-life care outcomes:[1]

- Provided physical and emotional support to the dying person
- Used shared decision-making
- Treated the dying person with respect
- Provided family members informational and emotional support
- Provided well-coordinated care

RESULTS

- Most patients (92.1%) died in their "last place of care," defined as the last place where they spent at least 48 hours prior to death. 68.9% of patients died in a health care facility, and only 31.1% died at home. Of those who died at home, approximately 50% had hospice services at the time of death (Table 43.1).
- Informants reported that patients who died with hospice care had fewer unmet physical and emotional needs, were more likely to be treated with respect, felt the family was better supported, and were more likely to rate the quality of care as "excellent."
- Both nursing home decedents and decedents who died at home with home nursing services were reported to have higher unmet needs for pain.
- Families of nursing home residents reported greater concern regarding whether their loved one was treated with respect.

Criticisms and Limitations:

- The fact that information was not obtained directly from patients may limit the interpretation of these findings.
- The most appropriate timing for after death interviews is not known.[2] Most interviews in this study occurred between 9 to 15 months after a patient's death, introducing the potential for recall bias.
- Location of death may reflect many potentially confounding factors, including patient preference, patient/family caregiving capacity, severity of symptoms, and other psychosocial or socioeconomic factors.
- Hispanic and African American informants were less likely to be interviewed and are thus underrepresented in this study.

Other Relevant Studies and Information:

- All else being equal, patients prefer to die at home, though their preferences do not always correlate with death at their preferred site.[4]
- Recent evidence in a Medicare population suggests a trend toward more transitions of care in the last 90 days of life and higher rates of ICU use.[5] The same study also shows higher hospice enrolment rates, although more patients accessed hospice at the general inpatient level and used hospice for ≤3 days.[5]
- A previous literature review has shown that patients have improved pain and symptom management in nursing homes with a hospice presence, whether or not a particular patient receives these services.[3]

Table 43.1. Summary of Study's Key Findings

Outcome	Total % (Unadj., 95% CI)	Home with Home Care % (Unadj.)	Home with Home Care Adj. OR (95% CI)	Home with Hospice % (Unadj.)	Home with Hospice Adj. OR (95% CI)	Nursing Home % (Unadj.)	Nursing Home Adj. OR (95% CI)	Hospital % (Unadj.)	Hospital Adj. OR (95% CI)
Patient did not get enough help with pain	24.2 (21.1–27.3)	42.6	1.6 (1.1–2.0)	18.3	Ref	31.8	1.6 (1.0–2.2)	19.3	1.2 (0.3–1.9)
Patient did not get enough emotional support	50.2 (44.4–56.0)	70.0	2.7 (1.7–3.1)	34.6	Ref	56.2	1.3 (1.1–1.5)	51.7	1.3 (1.0–1.6)
Not always treated with respect	21.1 (18.3–23.9)	15.5	2.9 (1.5–4.3)	3.8	Ref	31.8	2.6 (2.3–2.9)	20.4	3.0 (2.2–3.8)
Family concerns about emotional support	34.6 (31.5–37.8)	45.4	1.6 (1.0–1.9)	21.1	Ref	36.4	1.6 (1.3–1.9)	38.4	1.5 (1.3–1.8)
Family concerns about information needs while patient was dying	29.2 (22.3–26.1)	31.5	0.9 (0.4–1.8)	29.2	Ref	44.3	1.5 (1.2–1.7)	50.0	1.4 (1.1–1.6)
Overall assessment of care as "excellent"	49.4 (45.9–52.9)	46.5	0.4 (0.2–0.8)	70.7	Ref	41.6	0.4 (0.3–0.6)	46.8	0.6 (0.3–0.7)

NOTE: Unadj. = unadjusted; CI = confidence interval; Adj. OR = adjusted odds ratio; Ref = Reference.

- Another study suggests that family proxies feel patients are more likely to get "excellent" EOL care and to die in their preferred location if they receive >3 days of hospice.[6]

Summary and Implications: This study characterized the quality of the dying experience in America based on place of death. Many patients at EOL and their families had unmet physical, emotional, or informational needs, and those who received dedicated home hospice services reported a better dying experience than who who did not. These results are bolstered by findings in other, more recent studies showing that hospice use improves perceptions among caretakers of the quality of EOL care.

CLINICAL CASE: WHICH LOCATION OF DEATH IS ASSOCIATED WITH THE BEST QUALITY OF LIFE AT THE END OF LIFE?

Case History

Mrs. Smith is a 78-year-old woman with metastatic lung cancer, chronic obstructive pulmonary disease, and cardiac disease. She received two lines of chemotherapy for her cancer but is no longer fit enough for cancer treatment. She prefers to focus on quality of life but cannot live independently anymore. She and her adult children are trying to decide where she will be best cared for at the end of her life.

Suggested Answer

Though there is no one right choice for all patients, most people prefer to die at home. Unfortunately, there are many barriers—access to hospice, adequate caregiving, appropriate prognostication, family support, and so on—making home deaths often implausible. This Teno et al. study demonstrated that patients who died at home with hospice services had fewer unmet physical and emotional needs, were more likely to be treated with respect, had better family support, and were more likely to rate the quality of care as "excellent." Additionally, hospice services independently improve quality of life and death for patients and their family members.

In assessing Mrs. Smith and her disposition nearing the end of her life, the following questions are helpful guides: Could her children care for her at home or pay for a caregiver? Does she live in a location with hospice services? If the answer to these questions is "yes," one could confidently recommend that caring for her at home with hospice would afford her the best care possible.

References

1. Teno JM, Clarridge BR, Casey V, et al. Family perspectives on end-of-life care at the last place of care. *JAMA*. 2004;291(1):88–93.
2. Lendon JP, Ahluwalia SC, Walling AM, et al. Measuring experience with end-of-life care: a systematic literature review. *J Pain Symptom Manage*. 2015;49(5):904-915-3. doi:10.1016/j.jpainsymman.2014.10.018
3. Stevenson DG, Bramson JS. Hospice care in the nursing home setting: a review of the literature. *J Pain Symptom Manage*. 2009;38(3):440–451.
4. Tang ST, Mccorkle R. Determinants of congruence between the preferred and actual place of death for terminally ill cancer patients. *J Palliat Care*. 2003;19(4):230–237.
5. Teno JM, Gozalo PL, Bynum JPW, et al. Change in end-of-life care for Medicare beneficiaries: site of death, place of care, and health care transitions in 2000, 2005, and 2009. *JAMA*. 2013;309(5):470–477.
6. Wright AA, Keating NL, Ayanian JZ, et al. Family perspectives on aggressive cancer care near the end of life. *JAMA*. 2016;315(3):284–292.
7. McPherson CJ, Addington-Hall JM. Judging the quality of care at the end of life: Can proxies provide reliable information? *Soc Sci Med*. 2003;56(1):95–109.

44

Liverpool Care Pathway for Hospitalized Cancer Patients

CARLOS EDUARDO PAIVA AND
ANDRÉ FILIPE JUNQUEIRA DOS SANTOS

The improvement in the end-of-life care was small after implementation of the Liverpool Care Pathway in general medicine hospital wards.
—COSTANTINI ET AL.[1]

Research Question: Is the implementation of the Liverpool Care Pathway (LCP) program effective in improving the quality of end-of-life care of patients dying in general medicine hospital wards?

Funding: Italian Ministry of Health and Maruzza Lefebvre D'Ovidio Foundation-Onlus.

Year Study Began: 2009.

Year Study Published: 2013.

Study Location: 16 Italian general medicine hospital wards.

Who Was Studied: Adults who died from cancer.

Who Was Excluded: Patients who were relatives of a doctor or a nurse working in the studied hospital.

How Many Patients: 308

Study Overview: This study is a cluster randomized controlled trial in which pairs of general medicine hospital wards were stratified by region, matched for assessment period, and randomly assigned to implement the LCP-I program (Italian version of a continuous quality improvement program for end-of-life care) or to follow standard health care practice (Figure 44.1).

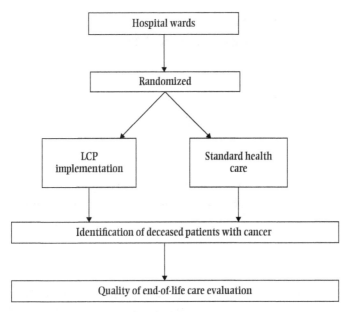

Figure 44.1 Summary of study design.

Study Intervention: General medicine hospital wards were randomly assigned to implement the LCP-I program or usual care.

Patients' family members were interviewed months after the patient's death. The interview included questions from the multidimensional Toolkit After-Death Family Interview (Toolkit scale)[2] and the Italian version of the Views of Informal Carers—Evaluation of Services (VOICES).[3,4]

Follow-up: 6 months.

Endpoints: Primary endpoint: the mean overall rating score on the Toolkit survey. Secondary endpoints: other Toolkit scale domains, namely, informing and making decisions; advanced care planning; respect, dignity, and kindness; family emotional support; coordination of care; and family self-efficacy.

RESULTS

See Table 44.1 for a summary of the study's key findings.

Table 44.1. Summary of Study's Key Findings

Quality of Care	LCP-I Wards (n = 119) Mean	Control Wards (n = 113) Mean	Difference Mean	P Value	Effect Size
Overall score	70.5	63.0	7.6	0.19	0.33
Informing and making decisions	73.5	64.3	9.2	0.08	0.31
Respect, dignity, and kindness	78.8	70.4	8.4	0.04	0.28
Family emotional support	46.6	38.6	8.1	0.20	0.29
Coordination of care	81.4	76.8	4.5	0.30	0.19
Family self-efficacy	48.9	44.4	4.5	0.36	0.16
Symptom Control	**n (%)**	**n (%)**	**OR**	**P Value**	**Effect Size**
Pain	100 (70.7)	89 (65.0)	1.3	0.46	NA
Breathlessness	108 (54.4)	97 (36.9)	2.0	0.03	NA
Nausea or vomiting	102 (83.9)	91 (77.2)	1.5	0.25	NA

NOTE: Liverpool Care Pathway, Italian version; OR = odds ratio.

Criticisms and Limitations:

- Clinical staff were not blinded to group assignment, which could have biased the results.
- There was a higher proportion of refusals by family members and a lower proportion of face-to-face interviews in the control wards. In addition, there was wide variability in the implementation process among the 8 hospitals. Only 34% of the participants (range 14% to 75% on individual wards) were cared for in accordance with the care pathway as planned.
- The study was underpowered, only enrolling approximately 80% of the planned hospital wards and patients.

Other Relevant Studies and Information:

- Previous research has suggested that the LCP-I program reduces the gap in the quality of care between hospices and hospitals by up to 27.5%: on an overall Toolkit scale ranging from 0 to 100, hospices were rated 90, LCP-I 70.5, and hospitals 63.

- In July 2013, an independent review of the LCP in the UK recommended that the LCP should be abolished, a recommendation that the UK government accepted.[5]

Summary and Implications: The results of this pragmatic cluster trial failed to demonstrate substantial improvements in the quality of end-of-life care for the LCP-I program relative to usual care. Of the 9 secondary outcomes reported by family members, only 2 showed significant improvements: "respect, dignity, and kindness" and the control of breathlessness. The program has now been ended by the UK government.

CLINICAL CASE: WHAT SHOULD THIS HOSPITAL CEO DO TO IMPROVE OVERALL QUALITY OF END-OF-LIFE CARE?

Case History

One hospital CEO identified end-of-life care as an important aspect of his institution, but such care was less than desirable. Regarding how to solve this problem, he questioned whether to introduce the LCP into his institution or to create a palliative care department. The LCP program for dying patients[6] was developed during the late 1990s in the UK and aiming to bring the principles of hospice care to general hospital wings.

Initially, when he became aware of the LCP, the idea of implantation seemed quite advantageous because he could use the same physical and human resources already available. However, what evidence supported the effectiveness of the LCP implementation?

Suggested Answer

In terms of scientific evidence, at the moment only one randomized clinical trial has been conducted to assess the impact of LCP implantation in a general hospital.[1] In this study, although some benefit was realized, the results were essentially negative, since the primary objective of the study, which was to improve the overall quality of end-of-life care, was not achieved. In contrast, multiple studies have found that specialized palliative care teams were associated with improved quality of end-of-life care. Based on the available evidence, the hospital CEO should invest in an interdisciplinary palliative care team and open a palliative care unit in his hospital, not implement the LCP.

References

1. Costantini M, Romoli V, Leo S Di, et al. Liverpool Care Pathway for patients with cancer in hospital: a cluster randomised trial. *Lancet.* 2014;383(9913):226–237. doi:10.1016/S0140-6736(13)61725-0

2. Teno JM, Clarridge B, Casey V, Edgman-Levitan S, Fowler J. Validation of Toolkit After-Death Bereaved Family Member Interview. *J Pain Symptom Manage.* 2001;22(3):752–758. http://www.ncbi.nlm.nih.gov/pubmed/11532588.

3. Addington-Hall J, Walker L, Jones C, Karlsen S, McCarthy M. A randomised controlled trial of postal versus interviewer administration of a questionnaire measuring satisfaction with, and use of, services received in the year before death. *J Epidemiol Community Health.* 1998;52(12):802–807. http://www.ncbi.nlm.nih.gov/pubmed/10396521

4. Costantini M, Beccaro M, Merlo F, ISDOC Study Group. The last three months of life of Italian cancer patients: methods, sample characteristics and response rate of the Italian Survey of the Dying of Cancer (ISDOC). *Palliat Med.* 2005;19(8):628–638. http://www.ncbi.nlm.nih.gov/pubmed/16450880

5. UK Department of Health. Review of Liverpool Care Pathway for dying patients. https://www.gov.uk/government/publications/review-of-liverpool-care-pathway-for-dying-patients

6. Ellershaw J, Ward C. Care of the dying patient: the last hours or days of life. *BMJ.* 2003;326(7379):30–34. http://www.ncbi.nlm.nih.gov/pubmed/12511460

45

Palliative Sedation Therapy and Survival

JOSEPH ARTHUR

> Palliative sedation therapy does not shorten life when used to relieve refractory symptoms.
>
> —MALTONI ET AL.[1]

Research Question: Does palliative sedation therapy hasten death?

Funding: Istituto Oncologico Romagnolo, Forlì and Istituto Scientifico. Romagnolo per lo Studio e la Cura dei Tumori.

Year Study Began: 2005.

Year Study Published: 2009.

Study Location: 4 hospices in the Emilia–Romagna region, Italy.

Who Was Studied: Patients with advanced cancer admitted to hospices for uncontrolled physical symptoms, psychosocial distress, or due to the terminal phase of their disease.

Who Was Excluded: Not indicated.

How Many Patients: 518.

Study Overview: This was a multicenter, prospective, observational, nonrandomized population-based study (Figure 45.1). Participants with refractory symptoms were enrolled into 2 cohorts based on the type of treatment they received. Cohort A included patients who received palliative sedation therapy (PST) and cohort B consisted of those who did not. Both cohorts were matched for gender, age class (≤65 and >65 years), reason for admission (psychosocial, uncontrolled symptoms, and terminal phase), and Karnofsky performance status.

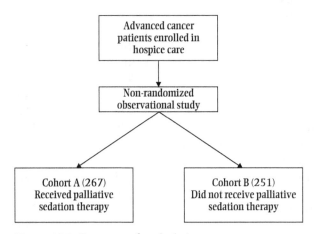

Figure 45.1 Summary of study design.

Study Intervention: The intervention was PST, which was defined as the use of sedative medications to relieve intolerable suffering from refractory symptoms by reducing the patient's level of consciousness. Refractory symptoms were defined as those "for which all possible treatments have failed, or it is estimated that no methods are available for palliation within the time frame and the risk–benefit ratio that the patient can tolerate."[2]

Follow-up: 22 months.

Endpoint: The primary outcome was overall survival. The secondary outcome was the overall survival of the two cohorts classified into subgroups based on the Palliative Prognostic (PaP) score. Survival time was calculated as the number of full days from the last hospice admission to the date of death from any cause.

RESULTS

- 25.1% of all patients admitted to the participating hospices received PST.
- The highest symptom indication for PST was delirium and/or agitation and the most common medication used for PST was neuroleptics (Table 45.1).

Table 45.1. SUMMARY OF KEY FINDINGS IN THE PST GROUP

Variable	Cohort A (PST)	
	n	%
Type of Sedation		
Proportional	234	87.6
Sudden	33	12.4
Mild	166	62.2
Deep	101	37.8
Intermittent	150	56.2
Continuous	117	43.8
Primary	229	85.8
Secondary	38	14.2
Drugs Administered for Sedation		
Neuroleptics[a]	161	60.6
Benzodiazepines[b]	145	54.3
Opioids[c]	68	25.5
Antihistamines[d]	63	23.6
Others	11	4.1
Duration of Sedation (Days)		
Mean value (SD)	4.0 (6.0)	
Median value (range)	2.0 (0–43)	
Refractory Symptom		
Delirium and/or agitation	210	78.7
Dyspnea	52	19.5
Pain	30	11.2
Psychological and physical distress	50	18.7
Only psychological distress	16	6
Vomiting	12	4.5
Other	10	3.7
Number of Refractory Symptoms		
1	168	62.9
2	89	33.3
≤3	9	3.8

NOTE: PST = palliative sedation therapy; SD = standard deviation.

[a] Chlorpromazine and haloperidol. [b] Lorazepam, midazolam, and diazepam. [c] Morphine. [d] Promethazine.

- The median patient survival was 9 days (90% confidence interval [CI] 8–10) in the routine hospice care group (cohort B) and 12 days (90% CI 10–14) (log rank = 0.95, P = 0.330) in the PST group (cohort A) (unadjusted hazard ratio [HR] = 0.92; 90% CI 0.80–1.06; adjusted HR = 0.86; 90% CI 0.74–1.00).
- The overall survival was not statistically different even after subcategorizing participants according to the PaP score: median overall survival (90% CI) in PST group (cohort A): 25 (16–26), 12 (10–15), and 5 (4–8) days; routine hospice care (cohort B): 27 (13–40), 11 (8–14), and 4 (4–6) days for PaP score groups A, B, and C, respectively.

Criticisms and Limitations:

- Physicians were allowed to use any sedation medication or procedure of their choice (i.e., the PST was not standardized).
- The investigators matched the clinical characteristics in both cohorts in order to minimize the probability of selection bias, though unmeasured confounding factors may still have influenced the study results.
- The study did not measure the efficacy of the PST intervention in terms of symptom control and quality of life.

Other Relevant Studies and Information:

- In contrast to the findings of this study, most other studies suggest that benzodiazepines are the most commonly used medications in PST.[3,4]
- Two systematic reviews of literature regarding the effect of palliative sedation on survival similarly showed that PST does not affect survival in terminally ill patients.[3,4]
- The J-ProVal Study also did not identify an association between the use of palliative sedation and survival.[5]
- The European Association for Palliative Care (EAPC) recommended framework for use of PST endorses palliative sedation as an accepted and ethical practice in the care of selected patients with otherwise refractory distress.
- The EAPC, however, recommends due caution with the use of PST since inappropriate administration can result in harms that undermine the practice.[6]

Summary and Implications: This prospective, observational study suggests that PST, when appropriately indicated and administered to relieve suffering in advanced cancer patients with refractory symptoms, does not hasten death.

CLINICAL CASE: WHO SHOULD RECEIVE PALLIATIVE SEDATION THERAPY?

Case History

A 75-year-old man with metastatic non-small cell lung cancer and a prognosis of days to weeks is admitted to the palliative care unit for symptom control and end-of-life care. He has elected to focus only on the management of his symptoms and does not wish to be resuscitated in case of any cardiopulmonary arrest. He continues to report severely uncontrolled dyspnea, which has been refractory to all kinds of conventional treatments including maximal supplemental oxygen therapy with high flow oxygen, morphine infusion, steroids, and bronchodilators. His current situation is causing him and his family an unbearable amount of distress. The family is requesting that he be made comfortable but are concerned that any such intervention will interfere with the dying process.

Should this patient receive palliative sedation therapy?

Suggested Answer

The study by Maltoni et al. compared patients with a terminal illness and a limited prognosis who received PST with another group of patients with similarly matched clinical characteristics who did not receive PST and did not find any difference in terms of survival.

The patient in this case scenario has a terminal illness with imminent death and severe symptom distress refractory to conventional treatment. He meets the eligibility criteria for PST. Contrary to the perception that PST may directly or indirectly hasten death, this and other multiple studies have shown that this is not the case. Moreover, the use of PST in this case is justified by the "doctrine of double effect," which states that if doing something morally good has a morally bad side effect, it is ethically acceptable to do it provided the bad side effect was not intended. The intent in this situation is to relieve intolerable suffering and not to end life, although the foreseen bad effect may probably occur.

The physician will need to first discuss the intended treatment with the patient and family members at bedside and answer any questions or concerns that they might have. It is also recommended that he or she discuss it with other members of the interdisciplinary team involved in the care of the patient before initiating the treatment. In order to ensure appropriate administration of the treatment, he or she may need to use a standardized palliative sedation algorithm or guideline if one is available.

References

1. Maltoni M, Pittureri C, Scarpi E, et al. Palliative sedation therapy does not hasten death: results from a prospective multicenter study. *Ann Oncol.* 2009;20:1163–1169.
2. Cherny NI. Commentary: sedation in response to refractory existential distress: walking the fine line. *J Pain Symptom Manage.* 1998;16:404–406.
3. Maltoni M, Scarpi E, Rosati M, et al. Palliative sedation in end-of-life care and survival: a systematic review. *J Clin Oncol.* 2012;30:1378–1383.
4. Beller EM, van Driel ML, McGregor L, et al. Palliative pharmacological sedation for terminally ill adults. *Cochrane Database Syst Rev.* 2015;1:CD010206.
5. Maeda L, Morita T, Yamaguchi T, et al. Effect of continuous deep sedation on survival in patients with advanced cancer (J-Proval): a propensity score-weighted analysis of a prospective cohort study. Lancet Oncol. 2016 Jan;17(1):115–122.
6. Cherny NI, Radbruch L, Board of the European Association for Palliative Care: European Association for Palliative Care (EAPC) recommended framework for the use of sedation in palliative care. *Palliat Med.* 2009;23:581–593.

46

What Patients and Families Want to Know About Hospice

REGINA MACKEY AND KIMBERSON TANCO

> Most patients and families who are referred for a Hospice information visit know little about Hospice and have substantial information needs.
> —CASARETT ET AL.[1]

Research Question: What do patients and families know at the time of their initial information visit with hospice and what are their priorities for information?

Funding: Greenwall Foundation.

Year Study Published: 2005.

Study Location: Urban, not-for-profit, Medicare-certified hospice that provides care for >3,500 patients a year.

Who Was Studied: All adult patients and their families from consecutive hospice information visits who spoke English.

Who Was Excluded: Patients who declined to participate.

How Many Patients: 237 patients and families.

Study Overview: This is a cross-sectional interview study in which all patients and their families referred to a hospice information visit were asked to answer questions before the hospice staff provided information about the program.

Study Intervention: Patients and their families were asked to describe their understanding of hospice. This was followed by 8 questions assessing patient knowledge regarding visit frequency, hospice payment, practical support, continuity of doctors, available sites of care, availability of treatment, emotional support, and spiritual support. Patients and families were then asked how much information they would like to have regarding each of the aforementioned factors on a 3-point scale (1 = just what I need to know; 3 = everything) and were also asked to identify the 3 most important questions in deciding to enroll in hospice.

Finally, hospice staff described how the decision about hospice enrollment was made, specifically whether the decision was a patient-made decision, patient-made decision with advice from family/friend, patient shared decision with family/friend, family/friend made the decision taking the patient's wishes into consideration, or family/friend made decision.

Endpoint: Primary outcome: Hospice enrollment information priorities (8 categories)

RESULTS

- Of 295 visits, 260 patients and families were invited to participate (88%). The ones not invited had some distressing symptoms or were actively dying. Of the 260 invited patients, 237 completed the interview.
- Interviews were conducted with the patient and a family member present (43%), with the family only (44%), and with patient only (13%).
- At the beginning of the study, 40% of patients and families (n = 94) knew at least something about hospice. Thirty-one percent (n = 73) could describe goals of care or services provided by hospice. Few patients and families were able to describe the role of hospice with respect to comfort care and symptom control (n = 27, 11%) or other hospice features, such as the role of visiting nurses, chaplains, or inpatient units (n = 11, 15%).
- Most of the patients enrolled onto hospice at the interview visit (90%).
- Family members made the decision in most of the cases (57%) because of cognitive impairment of the patient.

- Patients and families reported that hospice visit frequency, payment, and the level of practical support at home were the most important information about hospice for them (Table 46.1).

Table 46.1. SUMMARY OF STUDY'S KEY FINDINGS

Three Information Categories	% of Respondents who Selected the Item as One of the Top 3
Frequency of visits	60
Payment for hospice	59
Practical support	52

- Information about hospice care were categorized into 3 distinct factors: concerns about impending death (available sites of care, emotional support, spiritual support), concerns about practical support and assistance (practical support, frequency of visits), and concerns about changes from established patterns of care (payment for hospice, continuity of doctors, availability of treatment). Of these 3 factors, patients and families were most likely to select items concerning changes in care (83% selected at least one item in this category).

Criticisms and Limitations:

- This was a single-center study and may not be generalizable to other settings.
- It is not possible from this analysis to differentiative between the perspectives of patients versus family members.

Other Relevant Studies and Information:

- In a previous article, the author identified elements of care that contributed to positive and negative perceptions of hospice care in the last 24 hours of life. That study suggested 4 dimensions of the care that are more important in a family member's assessment of care: accessibility of hospice staff, continuity of hospice personnel, anticipatory guidance, and symptoms management.[2]
- In 2004, a study was conducted to evaluate the US dying experience at home and in institutional settings The results showed that bereaved family members of patient with home hospice services reported higher satisfaction, fewer concerns with care, and fewer unmet needs.[3]

Summary and Implications: This study demonstrated that patients and families have limited baseline knowledge about hospice. In making decisions about hospice enrollment, patients and families most value information regarding the frequency of hospice staff visits, payment for hospice services, and support at home.

CLINICAL CASE: WHAT DO PATIENTS AND FAMILIES NEED TO KNOW ABOUT HOSPICE BEFORE THE FIRST INTEVIEW?

Case History

A 65-year-old man with metastatic colon cancer has progressed through several lines of therapy and has no further treatment options. He has a colostomy in place and has lost 20 lbs over last 4 months. He has a performance status of 4 and his pain is under control with a fentanyl patch. His oncologist told him that his prognosis is in terms of months, and he recommends hospice. What should the oncologist ask and inform the patient and family about hospice before he is referred to hospice?

Suggested Answer

This patient would meet the eligibility criteria and would benefit from a referral to hospice. The patient seems to have a moderate symptom burden but will benefit from care provided at home particularly because his poor performance status may pose a burden to coming into the hospital or clinic for assessment and care. Hospice can continue to provide care for the patient's and family's physical and emotional needs, which may increase as the disease progresses.

The oncologist can start by asking what the patient and the family know about or if they had any direct or indirect experience of hospice. Basic hospice information such as baseline hospice nursing visits, hospice interdisciplinary team structure, and hospice insurance coverage can be provided. Further intricate details about hospice services may then be deferred to case management, social work, and the respective hospice representatives.

References

1. Casarett D, Crowley R, Stevenson C, Xie S, Teno J. Making difficult decisions about hospice enrollment: What do patients and families want to know? *J Am Geriatr Soc.* 2005;53:249–254.

2. Casarett D, Crowley R, Hirschman K, Galbraith LD, Leo M. Caregivers' satisfaction with hospice care in the last 24 hours of life. *Am J Hosp Pall Care Med.* 2003;20:205–210.

3. Teno JM, Clarridge BR, Casey V, et al. Family perspectives on end-of-life care at the last place of care. *JAMA.* 2004;291:88–93.

47

The Impact of Hospice on Mortality
of Widowed Spouses

KIMBERSON TANCO AND REGINA MACKEY

Our findings suggest a possible beneficial impact of hospice—as a particularly supportive type of end-of-life care—on the spouses of patients who succumb to their disease.

—CHRISTAKIS AND IWASHNYA[1]

Research Question: Does hospice use at the end-of-life reduce the mortality risk of the surviving spouse?

Funding: National Institute on Aging, Robert Wood Johnson Foundation Investigator Award and in part by the National Research Service Award from the National Institute on Aging.

Year Study Began: 1993.

Year Study Published: 2003.

Study Location: Source population drawn from Care after Onset of Serious Illness (COSI) data set, which was built from Medicare claims.

Who Was Studied: Spouses of patients (drawn from COSI) who died between their diagnosis in 1993 and December 31, 1997. The patients were diagnosed with any of 13 conditions (cancers of the lung, colon, pancreas, urinary tract, liver or biliary tract, head or neck, or central nervous system; leukemia or lymphoma; stroke; congestive heart failure; hip fracture; myocardial infarction).

Who Was Excluded: Patients with claims for the relevant condition prior to 1993.

How Many Patients: 195,553 couples with 155,638 widows and 39,915 widowers. 30,916 (15.8%) decedents used hospice care and 164,637 decedents did not use hospice care. Based on gender and propensity score, decedents who did and did not use hospice were matched resulting in 24,721 widows and 6,117 widowers matched as "cases" to "controls."

Study Overview: This is a matched retrospective cohort study comparing outcomes between the spouses of those who died with and without receiving hospice care services (Figure 47.1).

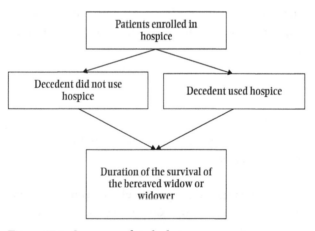

Figure 47.1 Summary of study design.

Study Intervention: Hospice use versus non-hospice use among the spouses of patients included in the study.

Follow-up: 18 to 78 months depending on when the decedent died.

Endpoints: Primary outcome: duration of survival of bereaved widow/ers of decedents who used or did not use hospice care.

RESULTS

- Of the 195,553 couples, a total of 30,916 (15.8%) of the decedents used hospice care before death (Table 47.1).

Table 47.1. SUMMARY OF STUDY'S KEY FINDINGS

	Male Decedents' Bereaved Wives (N = 155,638)	
	n (%)	Mortality rate in surviving spouse by 18 months (%)
Decedent used hospice	24,740 (15.9%)	4.9
Decedent did not use hospice	130,898 (84.1%)	5.4
	Female Decedents' Bereaved Husbands (N = 39,915)	
Decedent used hospice	6,176 (15.5%)	13.2%
Decedent did not use hospice	33,739 (84.5%)	13.7%

- The median interval between hospice enrollment and death was 22 days for men and 25 days for women.
- During the entire follow-up period from 1993 to June 30, 1999, 30,081 (19.3%) of the bereaved wives and 16,488 (41.3%) of the bereaved husbands died.
- Mortality rates at 18 months among bereaved wives was 5.4% among those whose husbands were not enrolled in hospice versus 4.9% among those who whose husbands had enrolled in hospice, with an adjusted odds ratio of 0.92 (95% confident interval [CI] 0.84–0.99) in favor of hospice use.
- Mortality rates at 18 months among bereaved husbands was 13.7% among those whose wives were not enrolled in hospice versus 13.2% among those who whose wives had enrolled in hospice, with an adjusted odds ratio of 0.95 (95% CI 0.84–1.06) in favor of hospice use.

Criticisms and Limitations:

- The study focused only on endpoint of death during the bereavement. Other endpoints among bereaved spouses, such as physical or mental morbidity or heath care use, were not studied.
- There is no clear rationale for why 18 months was chosen as the study follow-up time frame.
- Many unmeasured factors other than hospice utilization may have confounded these results.

Other Relevant Studies and Information:

- The National Hospice Study (1985) involving 1,745 patients and their families found similar rates of anxiety and depression among caregivers of patients who died in hospice versus at the hospital 4 months after their death.[2]

Summary and Implications: This population-based study using quantitative techniques identified a beneficial effect of hospice services on the subsequent mortality rates of bereaved spouses. It suggests that the type of care received by a terminally ill patient may have lasting effects for his or her family.

CLINICAL CASE: HOSPICE AS A NEXT STEP

Case History

A 65-year-old man diagnosed with metastatic pancreatic cancer, after surgery and several lines of palliative systemic therapies, has no further treatment options. He is bed bound with low appetite and has lost a significant amount of weight. The patient and his wife decide to decline further treatment and focus on going home and enjoying the remainder of his life with his family. The patient has a good support system, and the family is willing to care for him.

What would be the next best step for the physician to recommend to the patient and family?

Suggested Answer

Taking into account his current health condition and the probability of worsening of his symptoms as well as their wish to have him spend his remaining time left in the comfort of his home and with his family, a recommendation of home hospice care would be appropriate. The patient would meet criteria to enroll in hospice and benefit from such care. Home hospice services applies an interdisciplinary team approach to the care of the patient including physicians, nurses, social worker/counselors, chaplaincy, home health aides, volunteers, and/or other professionals such as physical, occupational, and speech therapists. Even with the interdisciplinary team, home hospice care requires a supportive home system and the help of the family and/or friends to attend to daily activities and care of the patient. In addition to improve quality of end-of-life care, hospice enrollment may potentially be associated with a lower risk of mortality in the surviving spouse.

References

1. Christakis NA, Iwashyna TJ. The health impact of health care on families: a matched cohort study of hospice use by decedents and mortality outcome in surviving, widowed spouses. *Soc Sci Med.* 2003;57:465–475.
2. Greer DS, Mor V, Morris JN, Sherwood S, Kidder D, Birnbaum H. An alternative in terminal care: results of the National Hospice Study. *J Chronic Dis.* 1986;39:9–26.

48

Attitudes and Desires of Terminally Ill Patients Regarding Euthanasia and Physician-Assisted Suicide

YU JUNG KIM

> Only a small portion of terminally ill patients seriously consider euthanasia or physician-assisted suicide for themselves.
>
> —EMANUEL ET AL.[1]

Research Question: What are the attitudes and desires of terminally ill patients regarding euthanasia and physician-assisted suicide (PAS)?

Funding: Commonwealth Fund, Nathan Cummings Foundation, American Cancer Society.

Year Study Began: 1996.

Year Study Published: 2000.

Study Location: Outpatient settings in 6 randomly selected sites in the United States (5 metropolitan statistical areas and 1 rural county).

Who Was Studied: Patients identified by their physicians to be terminally ill (expected survival time ≤6 months) with any disease and their designated primary caregivers.

Who Was Excluded: Patients with HIV, insufficient English literacy, hearing difficulty, or not competent to schedule an interview.

How Many Patients: 988 patients and 893 caregivers.

Study Overview: This is a prospective cohort study that interviewed and followed terminally ill patients and their primary caregivers. Twenty-four interviewers conducted interviews in person usually at patients' home. Follow-up interviews were conducted among surviving patients and caregivers of deceased patients (Figure 48.1).

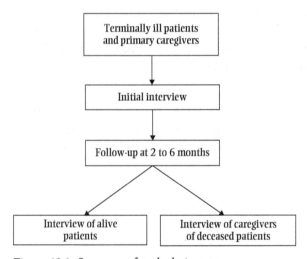

Figure 48.1 Summary of study design.

Study Intervention: Not applicable.

Follow-up: 2 to 6 months.

Endpoints:
- Attitudes of terminally ill patients toward euthanasia and PAS in standard scenarios
- Patient-expressed desire for euthanasia or PAS
- Stability of their views on euthanasia and PAS over time

- Hoarding of drugs for suicide
- Rates of death by euthanasia or PAS

RESULTS

- Among 1,131 eligible patients, a total of 988 patients were interviewed (response rate, 87.4%). In addition, 893 of 915 eligible caregivers were interviewed (response rate, 97.6%).
- In total, 60.2% of patients supported permitting euthanasia or PAS in a hypothetical scenario (Question: "When a person has a disease that cannot be cured, do you think doctors should be allowed by law to end a patient's life by some painless means if a patient and his family request it?").
- Only 10.6% of patients reported seriously considering euthanasia or PAS for themselves.
- Patients who felt more appreciated, were aged 65 years and older, and were African American were less likely to personally consider euthanasia or PAS (Table 48.1).

Table 48.1. SUMMARY OF STUDY'S KEY FINDINGS

Characteristic	Personal Interest in Euthanasia or PAS (%)	Multivariate OR	95% CI
All patients	10.6	–	–
African Americans	6.1	0.39	0.18–0.84
Age ≥65 years	8.3	0.52	0.34–0.82
Moderate or severe pain	13.5	1.26	1.02–1.56
Depressive symptoms	19.5	1.25	1.05–1.49
Feeling appreciated	8.4	0.65	0.52–0.82
Significant care needs	14.9	1.09	1.01–1.17

NOTE: PAS = physician-assisted suicide; OR = odds ratio; CI = confidence interval.

- Patients who had depressive symptoms, had more caregiving needs, and had moderate to severe pain were more likely to personally consider euthanasia or PAS (Table 48.1).
- At the follow-up interview, about half of the patients initially interested in euthanasia or PAS had changed their minds while almost an equal proportion newly considered these interventions.
- Patients with depressive symptoms (odds ratio [OR] 5.29; 95% confidence interval [CI] 1.21–23.2) and dyspnea (OR 1.68; 95%

CI 1.26–2.22) were more likely to change their minds to consider euthanasia or PAS.

- According to the caregivers of the 256 decedents, 5.6% of patients discussed euthanasia or PAS in the last 4 weeks of life, 2.5% hoarded drugs for suicide, and 1 (0.4%) died by PAS.

Criticisms and Limitations:

- Caregivers of decedents may not have been aware of all the activities related to euthanasia and PAS of deceased patients or may have been hesitant to honestly report cases in which patients died by euthanasia or PAS.
- Because only a small proportion of patients seriously considered or performed euthanasia or PAS, there was significant uncertainty in point estimates.
- This is a US-based study in which a majority of patients did not have euthanasia as a legal option. The study findings may not be generalizable to other countries or cultures.

Other Relevant Studies and Information:

- Euthanasia and PAS are increasingly being legalized and public support for euthanasia and PAS remains high (47%–69%).[2]
- More than 70% of cases involve patients with cancer.[2–4]
- Actual conduct of euthanasia and PAS is very low, and the majority of physicians oppose these interventions.[2, 3, 5-7]
- With the advance of palliative care and improved symptom control at the end of life, there may be a further decline in physicians' support for euthanasia and PAS.[5,6]
- Uncontrolled pain is not reported as the primary motivation for euthanasia or PAS in most studies.[6]
- Depression and psychological distress are consistently associated with interest for euthanasia and PAS.[1,5,8,9] Depressed patients are 4 times more likely to request euthanasia or PAS.[10]

Summary and Implications: This carefully designed prospective cohort study was the first to demonstrate that a small proportion of terminally ill patients seriously consider euthanasia or PAS for themselves. Furthermore, among patients enrolled in the study, interest in these interventions evolved over time. Patients with depressive symptoms were more likely to consider euthanasia or PAS and also more likely to change their minds.

CLINICAL CASE: HOW SHOULD PHYSICIANS RESPOND TO REQUESTS FOR EUTHANASIA OR PAS?

Case History

A 56-year-old woman with metastatic ovarian cancer has been treated with systemic chemotherapy for several years. Because there were no more standard chemotherapeutic options, her family has been seeking phase I clinical trials. Her performance status is now 3, and she has moderate abdominal pain and shortness of breath resulting from her disease involving peritoneum and pleura. Her pain improved with intravenous morphine. One day, while visiting outpatient oncology clinic, she politely requests euthanasia.

Suggested Answer

Physicians should openly respond to patients' request regardless of personal beliefs on the permissibility of euthanasia or PAS. Asking the patient to clarify why he or she is making such a request is an important first step. Physicians should carefully explore the patient's physical, psychological, spiritual, financial, and social issues influencing the request. Using routine symptom assessment tools such as Edmonton Symptom Assessment System may reveal unsuspected symptoms. The presence of delirium or mental illness impairing patient's capacity to make decisions should be assessed. Based on thorough clinical evaluation, comprehensive palliative care should be offered whenever possible.

As demonstrated in the Emanuel et al. study, physicians receiving requests for euthanasia and PAS should be aware that depressive symptoms and other psychological distresses can be significantly associated with these requests and that patients' requests can change over time. For instance, patients may have fears and concerns for future excruciating pain, losing control, or being a burden to their family.

A palliative care referral is clearly warranted in this situation. Giving patients the opportunities to fully express their concerns, reassuring that most symptoms can be controlled, and educating the patient on the dying process can be helpful in decreasing negative psychology and improving patients' sensation of well-being.

References

1. Emanuel EJ, Fairclough DL, Emanuel LL. Attitudes and desires related to euthanasia and physician-assisted suicide among terminally ill patients and their caregivers. *JAMA*. 2000;284:2460–2468.

2. Emanuel EJ, Onwuteaka-Philipsen BD, Urwin JW, Cohen J. Attitudes and practices of euthanasia and physician-assisted suicide in the United States, Canada, and Europe. *JAMA*. 2016;316:79–90.

3. Meier DE, Emmons CA, Wallenstein S, Quill T, Morrison RS, Cassel CK. A national survey of physician-assisted suicide and euthanasia in the United States. *N Engl J Med*. 1998;338:1193–1201.

4. Hedberg K, Hopkins D, Kohn M. Five years of legal physician-assisted suicide in Oregon. *N Engl J Med*. 2003;348:961–964.

5. Emanuel EJ, Fairclough DL, Daniels ER, Clarridge BR. Euthanasia and physician-assisted suicide: attitudes and experiences of oncology patients, oncologists, and the public. *Lancet*. 1996;347:1805–1810.

6. Emanuel EJ, Fairclough D, Clarridge BC, et al. Attitudes and practices of U.S. oncologists regarding euthanasia and physician-assisted suicide. *Ann Intern Med*. 2000;133:527–532.

7. van der Heide A, Onwuteaka-Philipsen BD, Rurup ML, et al. End-of-life practices in the Netherlands under the Euthanasia Act. *N Engl J Med*. 2007;356:1957–1965.

8. Ganzini L, Johnston WS, McFarland BH, Tolle SW, Lee MA. Attitudes of patients with amyotrophic lateral sclerosis and their care givers toward assisted suicide. *N Engl J Med*. 1998;339:967–973.

9. Suarez-Almazor ME, Newman C, Hanson J, Bruera E. Attitudes of terminally ill cancer patients about euthanasia and assisted suicide: predominance of psychosocial determinants and beliefs over symptom distress and subsequent survival. *J Clin Oncol*. 2002;20:2134–2141.

10. van der Lee ML, van der Bom JG, Swarte NB, Heintz AP, de Graeff A, van den Bout J. Euthanasia and depression: a prospective cohort study among terminally ill cancer patients. *J Clin Oncol*. 2005;23:6607–6612.

49

Factors Associated with Outcomes of Cardiopulmonary Resuscitation

DUTT MEHTA AND ERIC PROMMER

Predictive pre-resuscitation factors may supplement patient-specific information available at bedside to assist in revising resuscitation plans during the patient's hospitalization.

—LARKIN ET AL.[1]

Research Question: What pre-arrest factors predict postcardiopulmonary arrest mortality?

Funding: Not identified.

Year Study Began: January 2000 to September 2004.

Year Study Published: 2009.

Study Location: Database from 366 US hospitals participating in the National Registry for Cardiopulmonary Resuscitation (NRCPR).

Who Was Studied: Patients experiencing cardiopulmonary arrest (CPA) 18 years or older at hospital admission; those with pulseless cardiopulmonary (ventricular fibrillation included because it is a cause of pulseless arrests and would require defibrillation) arrest events requiring chest compression and/or defibrillation; those requiring emergency resuscitation response by facility personnel; those with a completed resuscitation record.

Who Was Excluded: Patients with events beginning outside the hospital, those who received treatment by non-hospital personnel, and those who had an implantable cardioverter-defibrillator.

How Many Patients: 49,130.

Study Overview: Patients and event data came from 366 NRCPR-participant facilities in 48 states and the District of Columbia and included 49,130 patients sustaining 54,651 cardiac arrests. This retrospective population database study involved (1) identification of preresuscitation predictors of CPA event mortality in hospitalized adults; (2) development of a multivariate logistic regression model for estimating in-hospital mortality; (3) prospective testing of the model on an independent validation set; and (4) quantification of the effect of important variables in the final model on hospital discharge survival outcome (Figure 49.1).

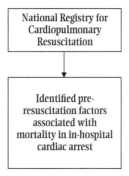

Figure 49.1 Summary of study design

Study Intervention: Not applicable.

Follow-up: Not applicable.

Endpoints: Primary outcome was in-hospital mortality. Patients discharged alive but with neurologic deterioration manifest as cerebral performance category scores of 3 (severe cerebral disability) or 4 (coma or vegetative state) were placed with nonsurvivors. CPA event outcome was defined by NRCPR as either event survival (return of spontaneous circulation (ROSC), sustained for >20 min with no further need for chest compressions or death. Any arrest that followed >20 min of sustained ROSC was defined as a new event.

RESULTS

- There were 54,651 cardiac arrests. Most patients did not survive the CPA event studied (55.2%). The vast majority died in the hospital (82.6%). One and one-half percent of CPA patients experienced significant neurologic compromise and were categorized with nonsurvivors (Table 49.1).

Table 49.1. PRE-EXISTING FACTORS ASSOCIATED WITH POOR CPR OUTCOME

Predictors of Mortality	% Died at Event	% Died at Discharge	Odds Ratio
Advanced age	59.1	86.4	1
18–39	52.9	81.0	0.67
40–59	53.2	83.1	0.78
60–79	60.7	89.1	1.29
80+			
African American	60.9	89.3	1.77
Noncardiac, nonsurgical illness category	60.0	90.6	1.0
Pre-existing malignancy	61.1	92.2	2.4
Acute stroke	55.3	89.1	1.57
Trauma	62.5	90.3	1.8
Septicemia	55.1	92.4	2.5
Hepatic insufficiency	53.4	92.7	2.5
Renal insufficiency or dialysis	52.8	88.6	1.7
General floor or emergency department location	50.6	77.3	0.40
Pre-arrest use of vasopressors or assisted/mechanical ventilation	58.1	91.6	2.43

- A total of 84.1% (82.6 + 1.5%) of patients had "poor outcome" by study definition. Availability of automated external defibrillators was not associated with CPA survival.
- Hospital mortality rate, according to the abstract, was 84.1%.
- One-half of events occurred in the intensive care unit (ICU).
- Almost all CPA patients had pre-existing conditions at the time of the event.

- Almost all patients had no documented CPA events prior to the index admission.
- The majority of pulseless rhythms were not shockable.
- High risk (i.e., >90% mortality) patients for poor outcome with CPR included older patients (68.3 years vs. 60.3 years); blacks (27.4% vs. 5.9%), and patients with non-cardiac–related illnesses.
- High-risk patients were more likely to be in the ICU (53.8%) with a high frequency of non-cardiac–related pre-existing conditions.
- 40% of high-risk patients were mechanically ventilated and/or were on vasopressors at the time of the event.
- High-risk events occurred longer after hospital admission (7.7 days) than low-risk patient events (2.6 days), indicating clinical deterioration with prolonged hospitalization.
- Good outcome was associated with beeper-dispatched CPR teams, events being witnessed, and patients requiring monitoring (outside ICU).
- NRCPR events occurring in general inpatient areas and emergency departments were associated with increased event mortality.
- Use of vasopressors, invasive airways (odds ratio [OR] = 1.55), and assisted or mechanical ventilation (OR = 1.40) were independently associated with mortality.

Criticisms and Limitations:

- The database may have missed data that could have improved the model's performance.
- NRCPR hospitals may not represent all US hospitals.
- Only internal validation of the model was conducted; that is, the model was not subsequently applied to a distinct patient population and assessed for its predictive value.

Other Relevant Studies and Information:

- Rudner and coworkers evaluated factors associated with survival in out-of-hospital cardiac arrests. Ventricular fibrillation as initial rhythm, arrest witnessed, and lay-bystander CPR and short time to defibrillatory shock was associated with improved survival.[2]
- Fischer and coworkers found that postarrest survival in out-of-hospital patients depends on short response intervals and life support being performed by well-trained emergency technicians, paramedics, and physicians.[3]

Summary and Implications: Identifying factors with poor outcome associated with CPR allows clinicians to improve their discussions with respect to do-not-resusitate orders. Clinicians can look to patient characteristics, pre-existing conditions, and ongoing treatments and convey risk for poor outcome to patients and families. This enhanced discussion can help patients and families choose care that avoids high burden treatments. Risk factors can be updated throughout the hospital stay as patient status changes, stimulating a continuing dialogue with patients, surrogates, and families.

CLINICAL CASE: WOULD YOU RECOMMEND CPR FOR THIS PATIENT?

Case History
You are asked to consult on an elderly African American male with rapidly progressing prostate cancer, sepsis, and worsening renal failure who continues to decline despite all therapies. The family insists on all measures be used to prolong his life. What can you tell the family about the success of CPR?

Suggested Answer
In this case the patient has several preexisting conditions that would lead to a poor outcome if CPR was initiated. Explaining to the family that performing CPR would have little success and likely cause harm may help them to reconsider this as an option for their loved one. Important predictors of in-house mortality include advanced age, pre-existing malignancy, acute stroke, sepsis hepatic insufficiency, or pre-arrest use of pressors or mechanical ventilation.

References

1. Larkin GL, Copes WS, Nathanson BH, Kaye W. Pre-resuscitation factors associated with mortality in 49,130 cases of in-hospital cardiac arrest: a report from the National Registry for Cardiopulmonary Resuscitation. *Resuscitation.* 2010;81:302–311.
2. Rudner R, Jalowiecki P, Karpel E, Dziurdzik P, Alberski B, Kawecki P. Survival after out-of-hospital cardiac arrests in Katowice (Poland): outcome report according to the "Utstein style." *Resuscitation.* 2004;61:315–325.
3. Fischer M, Fischer NJ, Schuttler J. One-year survival after out-of-hospital cardiac arrest in Bonn city: outcome report according to the "Utstein style." *Resuscitation.* 1997;33:233–243.

50

Influence of Survival Probability on Preference for CPR

CHRISTIAN T. SINCLAIR AND ALLISON E. JORDAN

Most older patients do not want CPR once they understand the probability of survival.

—MURPHY ET AL.[1]

Research Question: How does understanding survival probability after cardiopulmonary resuscitation (CPR) impact patients' preferences for CPR?

Funding: Not indicated.

Year Study Began: 1991.

Year Study Published: 1994.

Study Location: Denver, CO.

Who Was Studied: Ambulatory patients in a large, hospital-based geriatric clinic (mean age 77 years; range 60–99).

Who Was Excluded: Those unable to complete the interview due to dementia, psychiatric problems, or acute medical conditions. Also patients who did not speak proficient English, did not complete the interview, or did not return to the scheduled appointment to discuss advance directives were excluded. A total of 84 of 371 patients were unable to complete the interview process.

How Many Patients: 287.

Study Overview: This is a convenience sample of patients from a geriatrics clinic who participated in a structured interview during a general discussion about health care advance directives. The interview was conducted at the end of a routine office visit or scheduled as an individual visit focused on advance directives. The interviews were conducted by the lead author, a nurse practitioner, and 11 supervised medical residents (Figure 50.1).

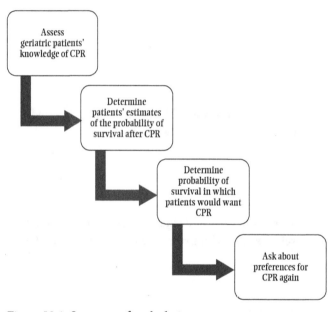

Figure 50.1 Summary of study design.

Study Intervention: Patients were first asked to estimate what they believed to be their survival probability after CPR in 3 clinical scenarios, as well as their personal preferences for CPR. The patients were subsequently informed of the likely survival probability based on multiple research studies.

Follow-up: This was a one-time study without follow-up. Nineteen patients were lost to follow-up indicating they did not come back for the interview and advance directives discussion when scheduled after a routine office visit.

Endpoints: Primary outcome: Preference for CPR after being informed of likely survival probability. Secondary outcome: Patient estimates of their survival after CPR in 3 clinical scenarios (accident, acute illness, chronic illness). The authors also attempted to assess the lowest probability of survival at which patients would opt to undergo CPR, as well as patient knowledge about CPR.

RESULTS

- Older patients were more likely to overestimate the survival probability after CPR.
- When patients understood the survival probability after a discussion with a clinician, many often revised their preference, with more patients changing from preferring CPR to not preferring CPR (Table 50.1).

Table 50.1. SUMMARY OF STUDY'S KEY FINDINGS

	Acute Illness[a] n (%)	Chronic Illness[b] n (%)
Patients who preferred CPR prior to knowing probability of survival	118 (41)	33 (11)
Patients who preferred CPR after knowing probability of survival	63 (22)	15 (5)

NOTE: CPR = cardiopulmonary resuscitation.

[a] Patients with acute illness were told survival was 10% to 17%. [b] Patients with chronic illness were told survival was 0% to 5%.

- Most patients in a geriatrics clinic estimated survival after CPR to be in the 10% to 40% range after either an acute or chronic illness.
- 20% (58/287) of older patients would choose to have CPR even with a survival probability of less than 10%.
- 25% (71/287) of older patients would not choose to have CPR, regardless of the survival probability.

Criticisms and Limitations:

- This was a single-site study of predominantly white Protestant patients and may not represent the diverse views of all older patients.
- The interviews were conducted by 13 different people without reference to reliability among interviewers.

Other Relevant Studies and Information:

- A systematic review and meta-analysis on advance care planning (ACP) in the outpatient setting showed the use of structured communication tools were better than an ad hoc approach in completing ACP, concordance of ACP preferences, future medical orders, and care received.[2]
- Discordant prognostic estimates are common in intensive care unit settings with surrogate decision-makers[3] and in oncology settings with patients and surrogate decision-makers.[4] The reason for discordance may be related to optimistic biases.[5]
- Code status discussions by attendings or residents in the hospital often lack estimates of survival probability and may be confusing for patients and surrogate decision makers.[6-8]
- In-hospital CPR rates have not improved from 1992 to 2005.[9]

Summary and Implications: This clinic-based interview of older adults demonstrated a wide range of preferences for CPR and a frequent overestimate of the success of CPR. After being informed of the true predicted likelihood of CPR success in different scenarios, patients were less likely to report a desire to receive CPR.

CLINICAL CASE: HOW SHOULD A CLINICIAN CORRECT MISUNDERSTANDINGS ABOUT CPR SURVIVAL?

Case History

You are seeing patients in a busy outpatient geriatric clinic. Your patient is a 75-year-old man who is here for a routine evaluation. He has a history of diabetes, heart disease, and osteoarthritis. Because you are an astute clinician, you ask about his advance directives and CPR. He replies, "Yeah, doc. I've been meaning to talk to you about that. I've seen it on television and I had a friend who got resuscitated and he turned out okay. I think I would want that. But I don't want to be a vegetable or a burden on my family." How do you respond?

Suggested Answer

The patient in this case has chronic medical conditions and has started to think about ACP, including CPR. Given his knowledge of CPR and personal experience, it is understandable that he would want resuscitation. However, it is not clear if he has a thorough understanding of what is involved in resuscitation and his chance of survival.

As the article by Murphy et. al shows, many patients have an incorrect idea of their likelihood of surviving after a cardiopulmonary arrest. When presented with information about their chance of survival in the setting of an acute or chronic illness, the number of individuals who still choose CPR decreases by 50%. A study published in 2015 found similar results when patients were shown a brief video about CPR.[10] Patients also have different thresholds for an acceptable chance of survival in which they would still want resuscitation attempted. Eliciting this information is important for discussions regarding goals of care.

For this patient, you may want to start the conversation by first asking about his understanding of CPR, clarifying any misperceptions, and then talking to the patient about his values as it relates to his quality of life. Once the patient understands all of the information, then you can help him determine if resuscitation is a reasonable option. The conversation does not equate to informed consent, as the patient is simply stating his preferences. However, knowing the patient's preferences may influence decisions regarding future procedures, which will require informed consent.

References

1. Murphy DJ, Burrows D, Santilli S, et al. The influence of the probability of survival on patients' preferences regarding cardiopulmonary resuscitation. *N Engl J Med.* 1994;330(8):545–549. doi:10.1056/NEJM199402243300807

2. Oczkowski SJ, Chung H-O, Hanvey L, Mbuagbaw L, You JJ. Communication tools for end-of-life decision-making in ambulatory care settings: a systematic review and meta-analysis. *PLoS One.* 2016;11(4):e0150671. doi:10.1371/journal.pone.0150671

3. Chiarchiaro J, Buddadhumaruk P, Arnold RM, White DB. Quality of communication in the ICU and surrogate's understanding of prognosis. *Crit Care Med.* 2015;43(3):542–548. doi:10.1097/CCM.0000000000000719

4. Gramling R, Fiscella K, Xing G, et al. Determinants of patient-oncologist prognostic discordance in advanced cancer. *JAMA Oncol.* 2016;174(12):1994–2003. doi:10.1001/jamaoncol.2016.1861

5. Zier LS. Surrogate decision makers' interpretation of prognostic information. *Ann Intern Med.* 2012;156(5):360. doi:10.7326/0003-4819-156-5-201203060-00008

6. Anderson WG, Chase R, Pantilat SZ, Tulsky JA, Auerbach AD. Code status discussions between attending hospitalist physicians and medical patients at hospital admission. *J Gen Intern Med.* 2011;26(4):359–366. doi:10.1007/s11606-010-1568-6

7.　Rhodes RL, Tindall K, Xuan L, Paulk ME, Halm EA. Communication about advance directives and end-of-life care options among internal medicine residents. *Am J Hosp Palliat Care*. 2015;32(3):262–268. doi:10.1177/1049909113517163

8.　Tulsky JA, Chesney MA, Lo B. How do medical residents discuss resuscitation with patients? *J Gen Intern Med*. 1995;10(8):436–442. http://www.ncbi.nlm.nih.gov/pubmed/7472700

9.　Ehlenbach WJ, Barnato AE, Curtis JR, et al. Epidemiologic study of in-hospital cardiopulmonary resuscitation in the elderly. *N Engl J Med*. 2009;361(1):22–31. doi:10.1056/NEJMoa0810245

10.　El-Jawahri A, Mitchell SL, Paasche-Orlow MK, et al. A randomized controlled trial of a CPR and intubation video decision support tool for hospitalized patients. *J Gen Intern Med*. 2015;30(8):1071–1080. doi:10.1007/s11606-015-3200-2

Index